# Ward
# Manual of
# Orthopaedic
# Traction

# WARD MANUAL OF ORTHOPAEDIC TRACTION

**Isobel Taylor** RN RPN OrthCert DipTeach(Nursing)

Lecturer in Nursing, Sydney College of Advanced Education
Formerly Co-ordinator, Orthopaedic Nursing Course, New South Wales College of Nursing

Churchill Livingstone

MELBOURNE EDINBURGH LONDON AND NEW YORK 1987

CHURCHILL LIVINGSTONE
Medical Division of Longman Group UK Limited

Distributed in Australia by Longman Cheshire Pty Limited,
Longman House, Kings Gardens, 95 Coventry Street, South
Melbourne 3205, and by associated companies, branches and
representatives throughout the world.

First published 1987

ISBN 0-443-03277-7

**British Library Cataloguing in Publication Data**
Taylor, Isobel
   Ward manual of orthopaedic traction.
   1. Orthopaedic traction
   I. Title
   617;.3    RD736.T7

**Library of Congress Cataloging in Publication Data**
Taylor, Isobel, RN.
   Ward manual of orthopaedic traction.
   Bibliography: p.
   Includes index.
   1. Orthopedic traction.   I. Title.   [DNLM:
1. Traction — handbooks.   WE 39 T243w]
RD736.T7T39   1987      617'.3        87-8017

Printed in Malaysia
by Percetakan Jiwabaru Sdn. Bhd., Bangi, Selangor Darul Ehsan.

# Preface

This book is written to help junior staff and staff new to the orthopaedic ward to approach the management of the patient in traction with confidence. Examples of common and not so common tractions are presented with a brief description of the mechanics and potential problems related to each set-up. Step by step descriptions of how to apply skin traction are accompanied on the same openings by photographs and schematic illustrations to add clarity to the text. Discussion of skeletal traction is confined to suspending and maintaining skeletal traction and preventing complications. Detailed discussion of techniques of application of skeletal traction devices and the orthopaedic conditions necessitating the traction treatment are beyond the scope of this volume. Readers are referred to the many available texts on the above-mentioned topics, some of which appear in the Bibliography.

It is hoped that an understanding of the principles and mechanics of the traction examples presented here will be transferable to any situation, however individualized it might be. Many set-ups are modified to meet specific patient requirements and medical preferences, however the principles remain the same. Considerable variation exists between individuals, hospitals and regions regarding the naming of some traction set-ups. An attempt has been made here to give a 'mechanical' name to each set-up followed by the common usage names in brackets.

My thanks are due to a number of people who assisted in the preparation of this manual. To my predecessor as Co-ordinator of the Orthopaedic Nursing Course at the New South Wales College of Nursing, Miss Marianne Garbutt, from whom much of the impetus and support came for the development of the format of the book; to my colleagues and students past and present for their valuable questions and suggestions regarding the text; to Misses Joan Carey and Brenda Simmons of the Children's Hospital, Camperdown, for their advice regarding the paediatric tractions and help, in conjunction with the staff in the Department of Illustrations, in the production of the photographs; to Messrs R. D. Hanssen and A. C. Macarthur of the Department of Illustrations at Concord Hospital, Sydney, for a large amount of photographic material; to Mrs Nora Collins for her painstaking care in producing the line drawings; to my husband, Brian, who critically appraised the manuscript and helped with typing, despite his own heavy commitments; and to Ms T. Shearwin, and Ms L. Fodor who completed the final typing. Finally, I wish to thank the publishers, in particular Judy Waters, for their great patience and forbearance in the face of the innumerable problems and delays I encountered during the preparation of this book. For any constructive criticisms or suggestions that readers of this manual might like to pass on to the publisher, I would be grateful.

Sydney, 1987                                                    Isobel Taylor

# Contents

# 1 Traction

Principles of traction
Classification of traction types
   Manual traction
   Skin traction
   Skeletal traction
Mechanics of traction
   Countertraction
   Position of the pulleys
   Vector forces
   Friction
Notes on traction apparatus
   Traction frames
   Bed and mattress
   Aids to moving and lifting the patient
   Weights
   Pulleys
   Traction cord
   Knots
   Useful adjuncts to traction equipment
General care of the patient in traction
Assessment of neurovascular status
   Circulation
   Movement
   Sensation

PRINCIPLES OF TRACTION

Traction treatment involves the use of a pulling force to a part of the body. Essentially, this pulling force overcomes muscle spasm and shortening, and in some traction arrangements, the effects of gravity are also overcome. By controlling movement of the injured part, traction enables bone and soft tissue to heal and can be used in a variety of conditions as a method of treatment. Its uses include:

— restoring and maintaining alignment of bone following fracture
— resting inflamed joints and maintaining them in a functional position
— gradually correcting deformities due to contracted soft tissues
— relieving pain due to muscle spasm.

As well as acting on limbs, traction can be applied to the pelvis and spine.

Traction can be achieved in several ways, though certain essential principles must be observed if the traction is to have the desired effect. These principles are:

1. The grip or hold on the body must be adequate and secure.
2. Provision for countertraction must be made.
3. There must be minimal friction.
4. The line and magnitude of the pull, once correctly established, must be maintained.
5. There must be frequent checks of the apparatus and of the patient to ensure that:

   a. the traction set-up is functioning as planned
   b. the patient is not suffering any injury as a result of the traction treatment.

Poorly or incorrectly applied traction can cause considerable discomfort to the patient and may retard rehabilitation. It is important, therefore, that staff responsible for setting up and maintaining traction are thoroughly familiar with the principles of traction so that the mechanics of each type of traction set-up are well understood.


CLASSIFICATION OF TRACTION TYPES

The grip or hold on the body is achieved:

1. manually
2. through the skin, or
3. through the bone.

## 1. Manual traction

Manual traction is exerted directly when the physician pulls judiciously on the part during manipulation to obtain closed reduction of a fracture or dislocation. Manual traction is also needed during the application of the traction set-up and during any adjustments to the set-up which necessitate the temporary release of the traction weight.

## 2. Skin traction

Skin traction is exerted in a variety of ways. Extensions, slings or splints are applied to the limbs; belts, halters and slings are used for the spine and pelvis. The grip on the body is less secure than with direct skeletal traction and the tolerance of the skin to weight traction is a limiting factor. It is utilised when shorter periods of relatively light traction forces are needed, for example with children and in the treatment of the upper limbs in adults and in the temporary management of femoral fractures or dislocations.

## 3. Skeletal traction

Large traction forces can be transmitted directly to bone by means of transfixing pins, screws and wire. Common sites are the distal femur and proximal tibia for forces exerted on the pelvis, hip and femur. The calcaneus site is used in traction on certain types of lower leg fractures.

## MECHANICS OF TRACTION

The mechanical components of traction systems are related to several factors:

— The way in which countertraction is effected.
— The number, angle and direction of the traction forces that are applied.

## 1. Countertraction

A pull in the opposite direction to that of the traction force is essential in order to overcome muscle spasm and to prevent the patient from being dragged towards the traction pull. This opposing pull, countertraction, can be achieved in two ways:

*a. In balanced (sliding, running) traction set-ups,* weights and pulleys are used to apply and direct the traction pull. Countertraction is provided by the weight of the patient's body aided by gravity when the bed or mattress is tilted away from the traction pull. Elevating the foot or head end of the bed on blocks is a convenient way to achieve

countertraction (Figs 1.1 and 1.2). When the foot of the bed is elevated, the head board can be raised slightly so that the patient's head
is not lower than the chest (see insert Fig. 1.1). Countertraction is
increased or decreased by further raising or lowering the elevated
bed end.

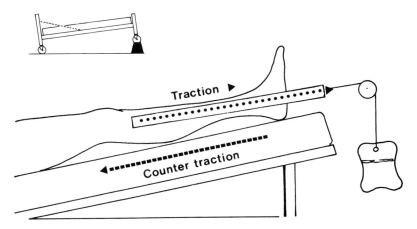

**Fig. 1.1** Balanced skin traction. Traction is exerted in the upper leg by means of skin
extensions placed on the medial and lateral aspects of the leg below the knee. A
spreader at the distal end of the extension carries the traction cord to the weight.
Countertraction is ensured by elevating the foot of the bed (insert).

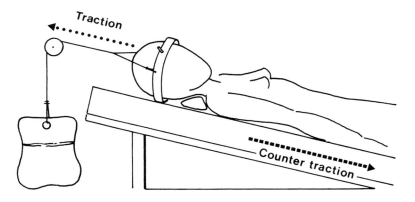

**Fig. 1.2** Balanced skeletal traction. Traction is exerted on the cervical spine by means
of a halo and pin fixation in the outer table of the skull. Countertraction is achieved
by the patient's body weight and gravity when the head end of the bed is raised.

*b. In fixed traction systems*, traction and countertraction are exerted
between two fixed points. An appliance such as a Thomas's splint is
used to gain purchase on the body at a point proximal to the muscles
in spasm. When the skin extensions on the leg are tied firmly to the
end of the Thomas's splint, the countertraction force is transmitted
up the sidebars of the splint to the ring encircling the root of the limb
(Fig. 1.3). In this way, fixed traction is a self-contained unit not

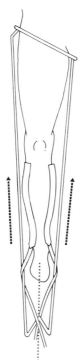

**Fig. 1.3** Fixed skin traction. Traction is exerted on the femur by means of skin extensions applied to the lower leg which are tied firmly to the end of a Thomas's splint. Countertraction is the force thus transmitted up the side bars of the splint to the ring.

requiring weights or bed elevation to achieve traction and counter-traction. Balanced suspension (Fig. 1.4) is sometimes added to the fixed traction system in order to elevate the limb and allow ease of movement in bed. Balanced suspension without traction (Fig. 1.5) is useful to simply elevate limbs in order to control post-operative swelling.

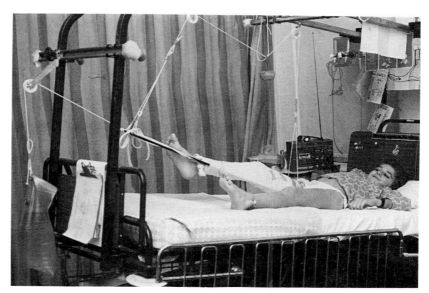

**Fig. 1.4** Balanced suspension in a fixed traction system.

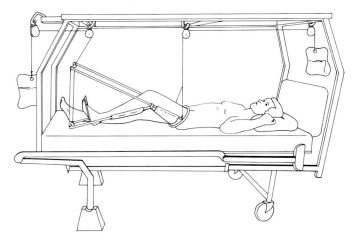

**Fig. 1.5** Balanced suspension without traction.

## 2. Position of the pulleys

The position of the pulleys on the bed frame determines the angle and direction of the traction pull. Once established, the line of pull is maintained and monitored by regular checking of the patient's position in bed and by periodic X-ray evaluation. The number of pulleys in the line of the traction force affects the amount of pull that is exerted. In single pulley systems (Fig. 1.1, Fig. 1.2), the amount of traction pull is virtually equal to the amount of traction weight applied. Where there are two pulleys in the line of the same traction weight, the amount of pull is almost doubled, because of the 'block and tackle's effect. This compounding effect is illustrated in Hamilton Russell traction where the amount of horizontal pull exerted on the leg is nominally double that of the applied weight (Fig. 1.6).

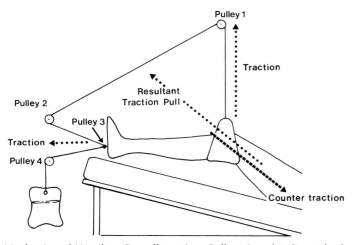

**Fig. 1.6** Mechanics of Hamilton Russell traction. Pulleys 3 and 4 direct the horizontal pull on the leg. The compounding effect of these two pulleys in line with the traction pull nominally doubles the applied weight. The vertical pull combines with the horizontal pull to produce a resultant pull in line with the long axis of the femur. Countertraction is achieved by elevating the foot of the bed.

### 3. Vector forces

By applying traction forces in two different but not opposite directions to the same body part, a resultant force is created. The direction of the resultant pull is determined by the position of the pulleys which direct the traction cords to the weight. In Hamilton Russell traction set-ups, vector forces are used to obtain a resultant pull in line with the long axis of the femur (see Fig. 1.6).

### 4. Friction

The presence of friction in the traction system cannot be eliminated. Friction gives resistance to the traction pull and tends to reduce the efficiency of the traction force. Therefore, it is minimised whenever possible. Ways of reducing friction in a traction set-up include regular checking to ensure that:

a. The pulley wheel runs freely.
b. The traction cord fits centrally in the groove of the pulley.
c. The weights do not rest against the bed or floor.
d. The spreader or footplate does not rest against the bed frame.
e. The mattress does not sag under the patient.
f. The bedclothes do not rest against the traction cords.

### NOTES ON TRACTION APPARATUS

### Traction frames

Frames vary in their construction to suit the various types of bed available. Consideration of the suitability of the traction frame is of great importance when obtaining beds for an orthopaedic unit. People familiar with the requirements of traction need to be consulted when beds are being considered for purchase. The frame should be one that is easily assembled and dismantled without requiring superhuman effort. It should be stable and secure and have sufficient overhead and cross bars and pulley attachments to allow for a wide variety of traction set-ups. The pulley attachments should be such that the cord and weights are able to hang clear of the bed ends. The components of the frame should be stored so that the parts are readily identifiable and accessible when needed. When in use, the frame should be checked periodically for movement and rattles, and be tightened or adjusted as necessary.

### Bed and mattress

A firm base is needed to provide stability for the traction apparatus. A good locking mechanism on the wheels is essential. The necessary positional adjustments should be available on the bed so that specific patient and limb positions can be maintained, for example, back, leg and knee adjustments as well as a tilt mechanism. The mattress needs to be firm enough to preserve good posture and alignment of the patient. A foam overlay or alternating pressure mattress on top of the firm mattress will help to protect the patient from decubitus ulcers.

*Side rails* are a necessary safety feature and of advantage to the patient in traction. They can be grasped by the patient when turning in bed — if turning is permitted — and while exercising. When lowered, the side rails should not impede access to the bed, especially during the lifting and moving of the patient. Side rails which reach almost to the floor when lowered prevent the people who are lifting from adopting a safe lifting stance, and put them at risk of back injury.

### Aids to moving and lifting the patient

The trapeze (monkey pole, patient helper) is an invaluable aid. The patient can grasp it to lift the trunk off the bed in order to ease pressure, as well as for the placement of bedpans and the facilitation of skin care by the nursing staff. The trapeze is attached to the traction frame at the head end of the bed. To obtain maximum benefit from the trapeze it should be:

— strong enough to support the whole weight of the patient
— positioned slightly anterior to the patient's shoulders
— adjusted to hang so that the patient can grasp it with the elbow flexed to about 20°.

In teaching the patient to use the trapeze correctly, it should be stressed that he or she should bend the unaffected leg, pushing down with the sole of the foot, not the heel, while pulling on the trapeze.

### Weights

Traction weights in a variety of forms are used: water-filled plastic bags, sand-filled plastic or cloth bags, or round metal weights on a weight carrier. The amount of weight to be applied is prescribed by the treating physician according to the type and purpose of the traction and the age and weight of the patient. The amount of weight is not normally altered without reference to the prescribing physician.

Too little weight renders the traction treatment ineffective; too much weight risks soft tissue damage and overdistraction of the fracture. The adequacy of the traction weight can be judged by radiographic estimation and by the use of a tape measure to compare the length of the treated limb with that of the unaffected limb. Weights are tied securely to the traction cord so that they hang freely. If a weight is hung above the patient, it must have a safety loop of cord attaching it independently to the overhead bar.

### Pulleys

The position of the pulleys determines the angle and direction of the traction pull. The number of pulleys affects the magnitude of the pull exerted. In a single-pulley system, the traction force is equal to the amount of weight attached. If there are two pulleys in the line of the traction force, the traction force exerted is nominally twice that of the amount of weight applied, owing to the compound effect of the pulleys.

The wheel of each pulley should run freely and silently. A squeaking pulley is not only irritating, especially to the patient, but is also less efficient. Periodic oiling of the pulley wheels will prevent such problems.

### Traction cord

The traction cord thickness should be compatible with the pulley size. Braided nylon cord 3–4 mm ($\frac{1}{8}$–$\frac{1}{4}$ inch) thick is generally suitable. If the cord is too thick to fit centrally in the groove of the pulley, the efficiency of the traction pull is reduced because of the friction generated. Traction cord should not be reused; it does stretch and weaken with use and can break. Lengths of cord should never be joined for use as a single length. The knots are a potential weak spot and could become jammed in the pulleys.

When several suspension cords are included in the traction set-up, it is useful to either use a coloured cord for the traction line or to colour the traction line cord, say, red with a broad-tipped felt pen. This identification of the traction pull helps to ensure that the traction line is not unwittingly altered during positional adjustments of the patient or equipment. The patient can also be taught to maintain his or her position relative to the direction of the pull.

## Knots

It is a matter of choice and expertise which knots are used to attach weights and appliances. Knots should be chosen according to their security, ease of tying and untying and the involvement of minimal lengths of cord. Although some common knots are illustrated here, practice is the only way to learn to tie knots. A simple overhand loop (Fig. 1.7) or a slip knot (Fig. 1.8) is suitable for weight carriers and bag weights. The clove hitch (Fig. 1.9) is a useful knot for attaching a cord to an appliance, as it is self-tightening and unlikely to slip. The barrel hitch (Fig. 1.10) can be used to attach a loop of cord to a single cord and is easily converted to a reef knot (Fig. 1.11) when the desired position of the knot is fixed along the loop. Half hitches (Fig. 1.12) are good reinforcing knots. On the other hand, elaborate 'granny' knots and square knots take up a lot of distance along the cord and are difficult to untie.

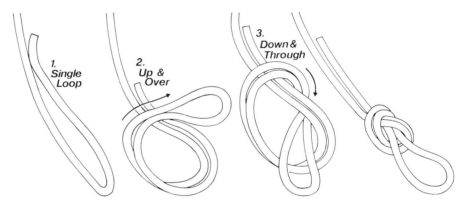

**Fig. 1.7** Overhand loop knot.

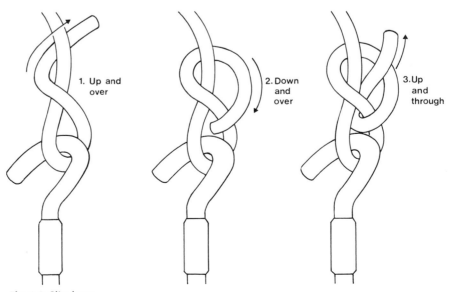

**Fig. 1.8** Slip knot.

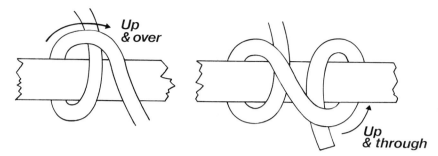

**Fig. 1.9** Clove hitch.

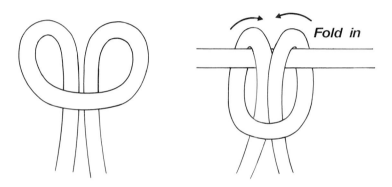

**Fig. 1.10** Barrel hitch.

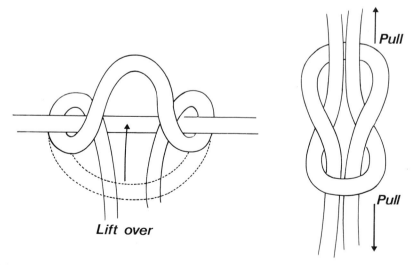

**Fig. 1.11** Reef knot.

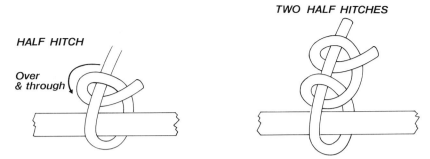

**Fig. 1.12** Half hitches.

After the traction has been set up and all adjustments have been made, the free end of the traction cord is taped to the cord above the knot with zinc oxide strapping to prevent fraying and to give added security. It is helpful if the end of the zinc oxide strapping is folded in on itself so as to leave a convenient tag which is easily grasped when the strapping is to be removed. The knot itself, however, should not be taped.

### Useful adjuncts to traction equipment

1. A goniometer is useful to check angles of joints and limbs relative to the mattress and traction cords.
2. A tape measure is essential for estimating the efficacy of the traction pull.
3. A hand mirror, modified with a long handle, and a torch are very useful for inspecting the skin for signs of pressure if the patient cannot be turned easily.
4. Angled mirrors, prism glasses and reading frames are essential aids for patients who have to lie flat for long periods.

*Storage of traction components* should be such that the component parts are readily accessible. A traction trolley, containing all of the small equipment needed and which can be wheeled to the bedside, saves time.

## GENERAL CARE OF THE PATIENT IN TRACTION

Adequate explanation of the procedures to be used in applying and maintaining the traction is essential to reassure the patient. If the patient understands what is involved in the procedures, he or she is less likely to be anxious about them and more likely to comply with the treatment. The thought of being literally tied to the bed for a not inconsiderable period of time is a daunting prospect for any patient and is, indeed, physically hazardous to an extent. The management of the patient is aimed, then, at maintaining his or her psychological and physical wellbeing and promoting an early return to a normal, or as near normal as possible, lifestyle.

In discussing with the patient the length of time he or she will be in traction, it is advisable to give an estimated time, rather than a definite one. Some patients calculate their time in traction to the very day and are bitterly disappointed when that day arrives and a decision has to be made to prolong the traction treatment.

It must be borne in mind that patients in traction may be suffering emotional, social and financial problems as a result of hospitalisation. Some may be facing the prospect of legal proceedings against them as a result of the accident that brought them to hospital. Early consultation with a social worker may help to avert depression and prevent a crisis situation developing for that patient.

Rehabilitation and discharge planning are best discussed early in the treatment. It may be that the patient will be left with some degree of disability, and contact must be made with the occupational therapist early in the planning process.

The negative physical effects of bed rest can be largely overcome by conscientious nursing care and good physiotherapy. In order to combat muscle wasting and joint stiffness, specific exercises need to be done regularly on a daily basis. Range-of-movement exercises to joints and static muscle-setting exercises to the affected limb, once taught to the patient, should be regularly encouraged throughout the day. Setting aside 'exercise times' and encouraging patients to exercise as a group works well in some units. If physiotherapy rounds are made at established times in a unit, it is essential that nursing and medical care is scheduled so that the physiotherapist can have uninterrupted access to the patient during that time, if at all possible. The specific exercises, with any special limitations to be observed, should be included in the nursing care plan, as should details of any restrictions on position and movement in sitting up and turning, for that patient.

Maintenance of optimal nutrition can be a problem if the patient's appetite is poor, or if boredom with the hospital food has set in. Again, adequate explanation regarding nutritional requirements necessary for healing may help, and early consultation with the dietician and the patient's family should allow solutions to be found.

Constipation is likely to become a problem because of the combination of immobility, analgesic intake and embarrassment at using a bed-pan. Adequate bulk in the diet and increased fluid intake should help in its prevention. Stool softening preparations and suppositories on a regular basis may be needed to establish a reasonable pattern. Ensuring privacy when the patient wants to use a pan may require the addition of portable screens if the traction apparatus is such that the bedside screens are not adequate. Slipper or fracture bedpans are more comfortable in some circumstances and can be slipped under the patient without too much disruption to their position.

It often helps the patient's mental outlook if the bed can be moved outdoors onto a verandah or even to a recreational area if one adjoins the ward. Children particularly enjoy the change of scene and benefit from the exposure to sunshine and fresh air.

Prevention of complications arising from the treatment itself requires regular checking and recording of the patient's neurovascular status. Any complaints of pain, tingling or weakness in an extremity should alert the staff to the possibility of complication; any signs of swelling, pallor or blueness in the skin must be investigated and the problem corrected.

X-rays are needed to check the position of the fracture and to determine the efficacy of the traction and the progression of the healing. If the proposed dates for these check X-rays are recorded prominently in the patient's case notes, there is less chance of a check X-ray being missed and not available when it is needed. A check X-ray is a wise precaution following any significant alteration or interruption to the traction pull.


## ASSESSMENT OF NEUROVASCULAR STATUS

Musculoskeletal trauma always carries the potential for harm to the surrounding soft tissues, particularly the neurovascular system. The injury at the fracture site may cause immediate damage or the subsequent swelling may be the factor that affects the integrity of the nerves and blood vessels in the area. Sometimes the damage is caused by the treatment of the fracture, for example, pressure from casts or excessive tension from traction. It is essential that the neurovascular status of the injured and treated limb is established and evaluated at regular intervals. The accurate recording of such information is mandatory for the protection of the patient (and of hospital personnel should legal proceedings ensue).

The length of interval between neurovascular checks will depend on the severity and type of the initial injury and on the observed status of the limb. As a general guideline the checks are carried out hourly for 24 hours following the initial injury, surgery, application of a cast or splint, or the application of traction. After 24 hours if there is no evidence of neurovascular compromise the checks are done every 2–4 hours. The checks consist of evaluation of circulation, movement and sensation.

### Circulation

Assessment of circulatory status of an extremity involves checking for colour, temperature, capillary refill in the nail beds, and pulses. On the upper limb the radial pulse is most commonly palpated. On the lower limb the dorsalis pedis pulse can be palpated between the first and second metatarsals on the dorsum of the foot (Fig. 1.13C). Another pulse which can be checked is the posteriotibial pulse (Fig. 1.13B). These pulses can be difficult to locate, particularly if swelling is present. If, at the initial check, the pulses can be palpated, the sites should be marked on the skin with an ink marker.

The temperature and colour of the skin may be influenced by the environment. The use of ice to control swelling or a wet cast will obviously have an effect, and such factors should be recorded on the observation chart.

Assessment of circulatory status does not rest on any one of these signs (pulse, colour or temperature) alone, but is evaluated on the basis of the combined information obtained and by comparison with the unaffected limb.

### Movement

Assessment of motion requires the active contraction of muscle groups below the level of injury. Inability to initiate active contraction of muscles may indicate compromised nerve function. The power of the movement should also be assessed and compared with the corresponding muscles on the unaffected limb. It is important to remember that reduced movement or power may be a result of pain or fear of producing pain.

In the lower limb, active dorsiflexion (Fig. 1.13B) and plantar flexion (Fig. 1.13A) can be evaluated by asking the patient to pull the toes up and push the foot down against the examiner's hand. In the upper limb, movement of the inside groups innervated by the radial, median and ulnar nerves are evaluated as shown in Figure 1.14.

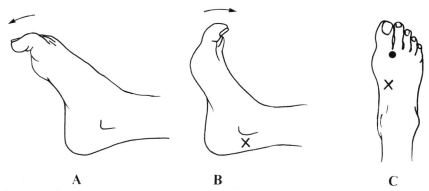

A        B        C

**Fig. 1.13** Neurovascular assessment of the lower limb. (A) The arrow indicates plantar flexion of the foot. (B) Dorsiflexion of the foot. The X marks the approximate site of the posteriotibial pulse. (C) The black circle indicates the area checked for sensation. The X marks the site of the dorsalis pedis pulse.

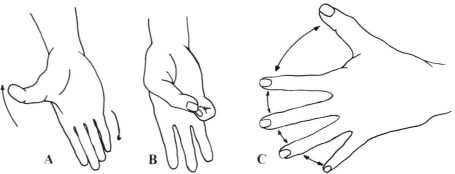

**Fig. 1.14** Assessment of movement of the muscle groups innervated by the three nerves supplying the hand. (A) Radial nerve: extension of the finger and wrist. (B) Median nerve: finger and thumb opposition. (C) Ulnar nerve: spreading the fingers and moving the wrist laterally.

### Sensation

Changes in sensation can indicate impairment of nerve function. The pattern of sensation change or loss provides information about the site at which impairment is occurring. Paraesthesias such as numbness, tingling, and burning type pain indicate a nerve's decreased ability to transmit impulses accurately. The cause may be due to the initial injury or subsequently as a result of decreased circulation due to an increase of tissue pressure. It is important to establish accurate baseline information so that later observations can distinguish progressive dysfunction.

Sensory function is tested by touching the skin lightly with the fingers or a sharp object, such as a pin. Sensation in the upper limb is assessed by evaluating each of the three nerves which supply the hand, indicated by the black circles in Figure 1.15. Alterations in neurovascular observation checks should not only be recorded accurately but trends of deviation from the baseline assessment should be promptly brought to the attention of the treating physician.

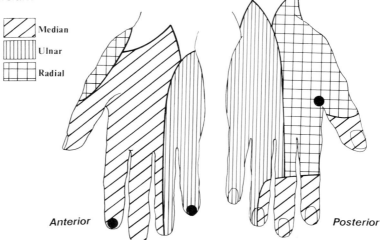

**Fig. 1.15** Sensory distribution of the nerves that supply the hand.

# 2 Skin traction

## LIMITATIONS OF SKIN TRACTION

Skin is susceptible to damage from large traction forces applied for more than a few days. Therefore, its use is limited to those instances where a relatively light pull or an intermittent traction pull is indicated. Weights generally do not exceed 4.5 kg (10 lb) for continuous skin traction. Skin extensions to limbs are applied on both sides of the limb leaving a strip of skin free. This prevents a constrictive, tourniquet-like effect occurring. When applied to a fractured limb, the extensions do not extend above the fracture site. Given these limitations, the extensions are applied over as wide an area as possible in order to reduce the intensity of the traction force on each square unit of skin.

## CONTRAINDICATIONS TO SKIN TRACTION

1. A history of a pre-existing health problem which predisposes the skin to damage and poor healing. Examples are diabetes, prolonged use of steroid drugs, neurovascular deficit, varicose ulcers, and peripheral vascular disease.
2. Any wounds, sores, abrasions or rashes in the area where skin traction is to be applied.
3. Any suspicion of impairment of circulation.
4. Marked swelling in the area.
5. A history of hypersensitive skin.

## TYPES OF SKIN EXTENSIONS

*Non-adhesive extensions* are used on fragile or atrophic skin. They consist of lengths of soft foam rubber, laminated to a strong cloth backing. The surface of the extension is covered by tiny holes for ventilation. Commercial kits are available in adult and child size, complete with foam padding already in place to protect the malleoli. Also included in each kit are a spreader, traction cord, and a retaining bandage (Fig. 2.1). The non-adhesive extensions rely on the friction of the foam surface against the skin and a firm retaining bandage to stay in place when the traction weight is applied. The grip is less secure than with adhesive extensions and the weight applied is usually restricted to 3 kg (7 lb). Frequent checks for slipping are required and reapplication may be necessary several times a day.

*Adhesive skin extensions.* These consist of one way (crosswise) stretch Elastoplast with an adhesive surface protected by a backing film. Commercial kits are available in two sizes, complete with foam padding, spreader, traction cord and retaining bandage. Hypoallergenic kits are available for people who are sensitive to zinc oxide adhesive.

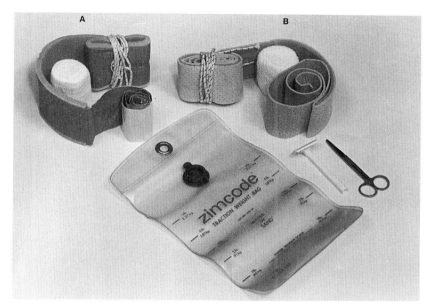

**Fig. 2.1** Commercial traction kits. (A) Adhesive Elastoplast. (B) Non-adhesive vented foam.

## MAKING SKIN EXTENSIONS

If commercial kits are unavailable or are of an inappropriate size, a set can be readily made using a roll of Elastoplast extension plaster.

**Extensions for a child in a balanced traction set-up, for example Bryant's (Gallows) traction.**

Requirements

- Tape measure.
- Scissors.
- Spreader 6.5 cm (2.5 in) with central hole.
- Traction cord.
- Extension plaster 5 cm (2 in) wide.

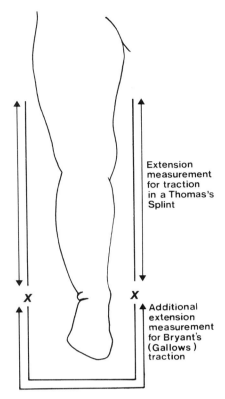

**Extension measurement for traction in a Thomas's Splint**

**Additional extension measurement for Bryant's (Gallows) traction**

**Fig. 2.2** Measuring skin extensions in fixed or balanced traction. For use in Bryant's (Gallows) traction the extension plaster is cut in a single length which extends from the lateral thigh around to the medial thigh. A shorter length which extends from the lateral to the medial malleolus is cut to make a lining piece (see Fig. 2.3).

Method

1. Measure the limb as shown in Figure 2.2. Estimate the required length of extension as follows:

    a. double the measurement from the thigh to a point 5 cm (2 in) beyond the heel
    b. add the width of the spreader.

2. Estimate the length of the inner lining piece as follows:

    a. double the length from the malleolus to a point 5 cm (2 in) beyond the heel
    b. add the width of the spreader.

3. Place the long extension plaster adhesive side up on a flat surface. Position the spreader centrally on the extension. Centre the short lining piece of extension plaster adhesive side down on the spreader (Fig. 2.3) and smooth down firmly (Fig. 2.4) to complete the extension (Fig. 2.5). Pierce the extension plasters over the spreader hole and thread and attach traction cord.

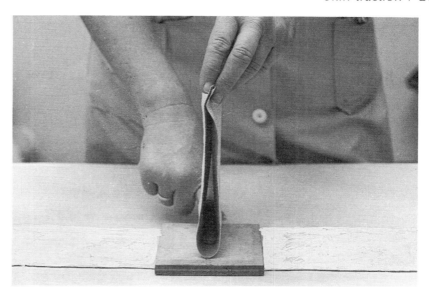

**Fig. 2.3** Making skin extensions for Bryant's (Gallows) traction.

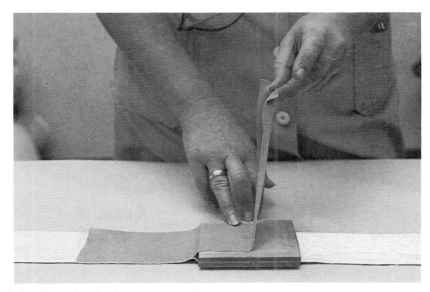

**Fig. 2.4** Centering the lining piece on the spreader.

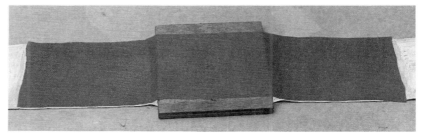

**Fig. 2.5** Completed skin extension.

**Extensions for a child in fixed traction in a Thomas's splint.**

Two lampwick ties 50 cm (approximately 20 in) long replace the spreader in this traction (see Fig. 3.18 p. 44).

Method

1. Measure the limb (Fig. 2.2) and cut two lengths of extension plaster.
2. Ensure that the extension reaches only to a point distal to the fracture level.
3. Attach the lampwick ties to the extension plaster by sewing them on securely as shown in Figure 2.6.

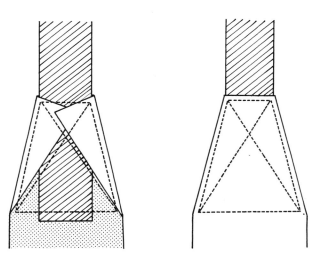

**Fig. 2.6** Attachment of lampwick ties.

REMOVING SKIN EXTENSIONS

Care must be taken to avoid damaging the skin during removal of the Elastoplast. Peeling the edges back slowly while pulling the skin taut is less damaging than pulling the extension off quickly. Some patients may need analgesia beforehand. A common regime for children is to first bathe the child, allowing the edges of the extension plaster to loosen. When the child is returned to bed the Elastoplast is gradually removed as tolerated by the child. Adhesive solvents help in the removal and cleanse the remaining adhesive off the skin.

## COMPLICATIONS OF SKIN TRACTION

1. Allergic reaction to zinc oxide adhesive can cause blistering of the skin. The patient will complain of irritation and burning under the extensions. Use non-adhesive extensions for susceptible patients.
2. Excoriation of the skin from slipping extensions. The limb needs to be inspected regularly to check for this, especially when the maximum weight is used.
3. Pressure sores over bony prominences are caused by inadequate padding of vulnerable areas. Check and change the padding as necessary. Check that the encircling bandages are not too tight.
4. Nerve palsy can result from pressure in vulnerable areas where nerves pass superficially to bony points. The common peroneal nerve over the head of the fibula is at risk in skin traction. The leg tends to roll into lateral rotation and may compress the nerve against supporting slings. Check the alignment of the leg routinely and assess the patient's ability to dorsiflex the ankle. The tendency to external rotation can be controlled somewhat by the correct placement of the skin extensions (see Fig. 3.6 p. 29), and correct bandaging technique (see p. 30).

# 3 Skin traction to the lower limb

Horizontal lower limb traction
  Buck's traction, simple traction, sliding traction, running traction
    Mechanics
    Requirements
    Application
    Variation 1 (Pugh's traction)
    Variation 2 (Extension boot traction)
Bilateral vertical lower limb traction
  Bryant's traction, Gallows traction
    Mechanics
    Requirements
    Application
    Potential problems
    Variation 1
    Variation 2 (Progressive abduction traction)
Two-directional lower limb traction
  Hamilton Russell traction, Russell traction
    Mechanics
    Requirements
    Application
    Potential problems
    Variation (Modified Hamilton Russell traction, split Russell
      traction)
Straight leg fixed skin traction in a Thomas's splint
    Mechanics
    Requirements
    Application
    Potential problems
    Variation 1
    Variation 2 (Straight leg balanced traction — Yale method)

## HORIZONTAL LOWER LIMB TRACTION

BUCK'S TRACTION, SIMPLE TRACTION, SLIDING TRACTION, RUNNING TRACTION

This is a balanced skin traction exerted via skin extensions to the lower limbs (Fig. 3.1). It is used in the management of conditions affecting the hip, femur, knee and lumbar spine when partial immobilisation and relatively light traction forces are required.

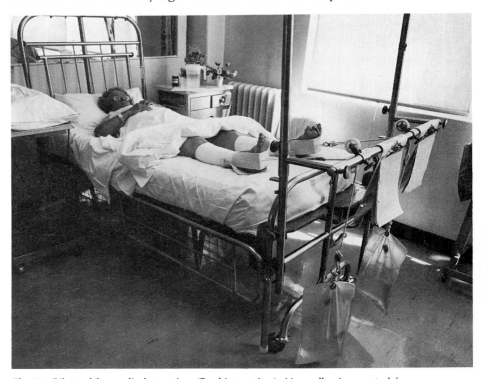

**Fig. 3.1** Bilateral lower limb traction (Buck's traction). Non-adhesive vented foam extensions are shown here bandaged to below the knee. The excess length of extension is folded back and secured by a few turns of the bandage. (Photograph courtesy Department of Illustrations, Concord Hospital, Sydney, New South Wales.)

Examples of its use are:

— in the management of low back pain, the traction being always bilateral in this case
— following reduction of a dislocated hip
— before and after arthroplasty of the hip joint
— to correct or prevent minor fixed flexion deformity of the hip or knee
— in the management of non-displaced fractures of the acetabulum
— in the initial management of Perthes' disease and Irritable Hip Syndrome in children
— in the temporary management of shaft fractures of the femur in children and adults.

### Mechanics

The patient is supine with the legs straight and in slight abduction. In a single pulley system, traction is exerted via skin extensions in line with the long axis of the limb. Countertraction is provided by the weight of the patient when the foot of the bed is elevated by 15 cm (6 in).

### Requirements

- An assistant to support the limb.
- Skin extensions of either Elastoplast or vented foam, depending on the integrity of the patient's skin.
- 1 or 2 spreaders, depending on whether one or both legs are involved.
- Wool padding for bony prominences.
- 1 or 2 traction cords, each 3 m (3¼ yd) long.
- 1 or 2 bandages.
- 1 or 2 pulleys, to be positioned on the frame in line with the foot (see Fig. 3.1).
- 1 or 2 weight bags, 2.3–3.2 kg (5–7lb) being generally sufficient.
- 2 bed blocks each 15 cm (6 in) in height to elevate the foot of bed (see Fig. 3.9).
- Tape measure.
- Scissors.
- Skin preparation materials.
- Zinc oxide strapping 2.5 cm (1 in) wide.

### Application

1. Position the patient supine with the legs extended and in slight abduction.
2. Record the neurovascular status of the limb(s).
3. Have the assistant exert gentle, steady manual traction on the limb (Fig. 3.2).

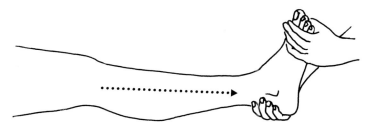

**Fig. 3.2** Manual traction is applied to the limb as shown by an assistant during the preparation of the skin and the application of the extensions.

A

B

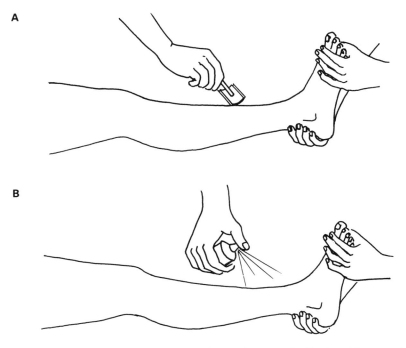

**Fig. 3.3** Preparation of the skin prior to the application of adhesive skin extensions. (A) If there is much hair on the skin, the area to be covered by the extensions is carefully shaved. Electric clippers are less likely to abrade the skin and are preferable if available. (B) The application of a semi-adhesive compound such as tincture of Benzoin enhances the adhesion of zinc oxide Elastoplast. This preparation is contraindicated however if hypoallergenic extensions are used.

4. Prepare the limb(s) according to the type of extension used (Figs 3.3A & B).
5. Cut the extensions to the desired length (Fig. 3.4). Foam extensions need not be cut, but simply folded back (see Fig. 3.1).
6. Pad over the malleoli, tibial crest and head of the fibula.
7. Before removing the backing paper pull on the extension — if adhesive ones are used — to stretch out creases due to the packaging (Fig. 3.5).
8. Tie a length of traction cord to the spreader.
9. Remove the backing paper while positioning the extension on the limb so that:

   a. the spreader extends 10–15 cm (4–5 in) beyond the foot to allow plantar flexion, and
   b. the lateral extension lies parallel to but slightly below the medial extension in order to discourage external rotation of the leg (Figs 3.6A & B).

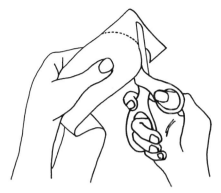

**Fig. 3.4** Cutting extensions. The Elastoplast tends to peel down at the corners. Rounding them off when cutting the extension to the required length prevents this.

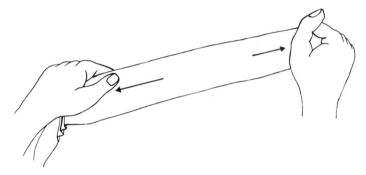

**Fig. 3.5** Preparing the skin extension. Before removing the backing paper from the extension, pull it taut to eliminate wrinkles.

**A**

**B**

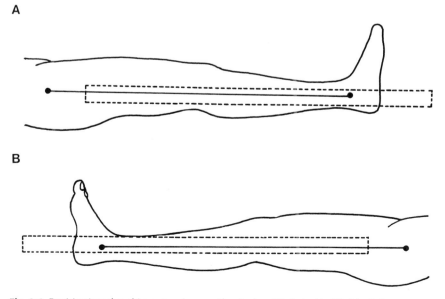

**Fig. 3.6** Positioning the skin extension on the limbs. (A) Lateral. (B) Medial.

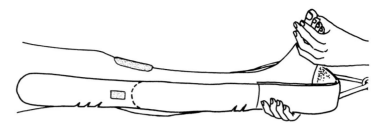

**Fig. 3.7** Padding the limb. The malleoli are protected by the foam incorporated in the extension. The tibial crest and the head of the fibula are padded (shaded area) before the encircling bandage is applied. (The broken line denotes the extent of the Elastoplast for below knee application.)

10. Cut small nicks in the extension plaster, if adhesive, at the knee and ankle to ensure that it lies flat and conforms to the contours of the limb. Ensure bony prominences are padded (Fig. 3.7).
11. Bandage over the skin extensions, leaving the patella free and bandaging from the outside to the inside of the leg to discourage external rotation (Fig. 3.8).
12. Pass the traction cord from the spreader over the pulley in line with the foot, and attach the weight (Fig. 3.9).
13. Tape the cut ends of the traction cord.
14. Elevate the foot of the bed on blocks if there is no tilt mechanism on the bed. Raise the head support so that the patient's head is not lower than the chest.

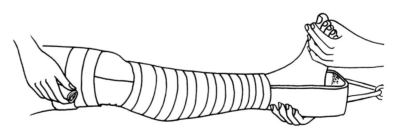

**Fig. 3.8** Bandaging. If above knee extensions are applied, the bandage covers the extensions but the patella is left exposed.

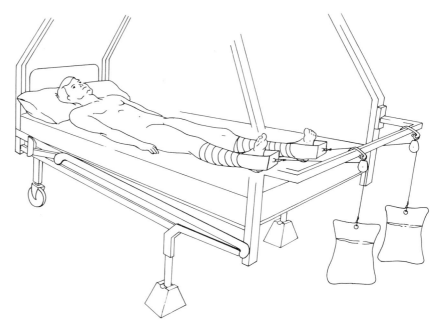

**Fig. 3.9** Completed Buck's traction. The traction cord is directed over the pulley in line with the foot. There should be enough room between the sole of the foot and the spreader to allow the patient to plantar flex.

### Variation 1 (Pugh's traction)

No weight or pulleys are used. The cord from the spreader is simply tied to the end of the bed or traction frame. The bed is elevated at the foot to provide countertraction.

### Variation 2 (Extension Boot traction)

In place of skin extensions a sponge rubber boot with spreader attached is available commercially. The boot reaches to below the knee and is open down the front for ease of application. It is applied to the bare skin and fastened over the front of the leg by several Velcro straps. Care must be taken to overlap the sponge edges to ensure that the Velcro straps are not in contact with the skin. Minimal forces only can be used with this traction as it tends to slip down causing pressure around the ankle. Frequent checking for slipping and for skin irritation from overheating is necessary. The traction boot allows intermittent traction only as it must be removed at least three times in 24 hours to permit thorough inspection of the skin, including the heel.

## BILATERAL VERTICAL LOWER LIMB TRACTION

### BRYANT'S TRACTION, GALLOWS TRACTION

This set-up (Fig. 3.10) is used in the management of femoral shaft fractures in very young children and in the preliminary management of congenital dislocation of the hip. Owing to the risks of serious vascular complications resulting in ischaemic fibrosis of the calf muscles or even gangrenous changes in the foot and ankle, it is only safe for children who weigh less than 16 kg (approx. 35 lb).

The contributing factors to the risk of vascular complications are:

1. The vertical position of the legs.
2. Tight bandages.
3. Hyperextension of the knees.
4. The amount of traction force exerted.

In children heavier than the limit stated above, the increased amount of traction needed to raise the buttocks just clear of the mattress would add considerably to the risk of vascular complications.

### Mechanics

Traction is exerted via full-length skin extensions to both legs. The child is positioned with the hips flexed to 90° and both legs are suspended vertically. The unaffected leg is always included to maintain the desired position and to facilitate toilet care. The knees are slightly flexed (Fig. 3.10). Enough weight is needed to lift the child's pelvis so that the sacrum just clears the mattress, thus ensuring that countertraction is provided by the weight of the child's body (Fig. 3.11).

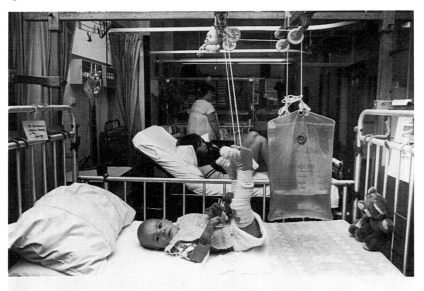

**Fig. 3.10** Bryant's (Gallows) traction.

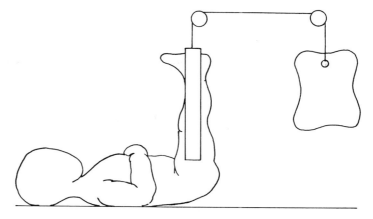

**Fig. 3.11** Bryant's (Gallows) traction. Countertraction is achieved by using enough weight to suspend the buttocks just clear of the mattress.

### Requirements

- An assistant to maintain the child's legs in the desired position.
- 2 sets of skin extensions including spreaders and bandages. If commercial kits are unavailable, assemble the extensions from extension plaster as previously described (pp. 20–21).
- Wool padding to protect bony prominences.
- Tincture of Benzoin compound spray or paint. Note that this is *not* used if hypoallergenic extension plaster is to be applied as it has a detrimental effect on the special hypoallergenic adhesive. (Check the advice on the box containing the extension plaster.)
- 2 traction cords, each 2.5–3 m ($2\frac{3}{4}$–$3\frac{1}{4}$ yd) long.
- 4 pulleys attached to the overhead bars.
- 2 weights of appropriate amount. Generally a total of between 0.5 and 1.5 kg (1–3 lb) is sufficient, depending on the weight of the child.
- Scissors.
- Tape measure.
- Zinc oxide strapping 2.5 cm (1 in) wide.
- A jacket restraint may be needed if the child is very active.
- Socks to keep the feet warm if the room temperature is cool.

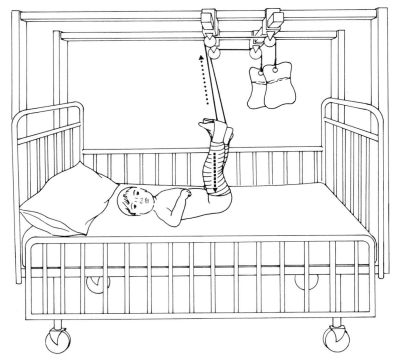

**Fig. 3.12** Bryant's (Gallows) traction. Positioning of overhead pulleys.

### Application

1. Position the pulleys on the overhead bars so that two are above the child's hips and two are towards the foot of the cot (Fig. 3.12).
2. Wash the child's legs if necessary and dry them thoroughly.
3. Check for any rashes, abrasions or hypersensitivity to Elastoplast. These are all contraindications to the use of adhesive skin extensions.
4. Check the neurovascular status of each limb and record it on the observation chart as baseline information.
5. Measure and cut the extensions so that:

   a. they come well up the thigh
   b. the toes just touch the spreader when the foot is flexed
   c. the extensions do not meet or overlap anywhere on the limb to create an encircling wrap. A strip of skin should remain visible down the front and back of the leg.

6. Tie a length of cord to each spreader with the knot on the outside.
7. If tincture of Benzoin is not contraindicated (see Requirements), lightly spray or paint the lateral and medial aspects of each leg.
8. Pad the malleoli with wool.
9. Have the assistant hold the leg so that the knee is in slight flexion when the extensions are applied. This helps to prevent hyperextension when traction is exerted.

10. Apply the extensions to the medial and lateral aspects of the legs, smoothing out any wrinkles. Cut small nicks in the extensions just above the malleoli and at the knee to mould them to the contours of the limb (see Fig. 3.7) and to allow movement at the ankle without friction.
11. Apply the bandages evenly at half stretch. They need to be reasonably firm, but must not be tight. Starting distally, direct the bandage from the outside to the inside of the limb to help minimise the tendency to external rotation (see Fig. 3.8).
12. Lift the legs perpendicular to the mattress, pass each cord through the pulleys and attach the weights securely (see Fig. 3.12).
13. Check that:

    a. the hips are flexed to 90°
    b. the malleoli are well padded
    c. the weights are hanging freely and out of the reach of the child
    d. the buttocks are *not* resting on the bed. There should be just enough room to pass one finger between the sacrum and the mattress; if there is not, add a small amount of weight to each leg equally until countertraction is achieved.

14. Tape the cut ends of the traction cords.

**Potential problems**

1. Impairment of circulation

This is the most serious complication that can arise because of the contributing factors described above. Therefore, a priority in the management of the child is careful observation of both feet throughout the duration of the traction treatment, but particularly in the first 3 days. A common regime is to carry out hourly checks for the first 24 hours, then 2-hourly checks for a further 48 hours, and 2- to 4-hourly checks thereafter. Both feet are checked for changes in:

a. colour
b. temperature
c. capillary return
d. pulse
e. active and passive movement.

There may be a mild deficit in colour and temperature, that is paleness and coolness, for the first few hours while the circulation adjusts to the vertical position of the legs. However, the nail beds should blanch readily on mild pressure and normal capillary return should be demonstrated.

The presence of pulse does not rule out ischaemia of the calf muscles, and in many instances, the pulse is barely palpable from the outset, so the estimation of pulse presence or absence is not reliable on its own.

Active movement of the toes is elicited by stroking the soles of the feet. Passive dorsiflexion should be full in extent and painfree. Painful or limited dorsiflexion is a reliable sign that the circulation is impaired and prompt action must be initiated. Such action includes:

- Alerting the treating physician.
- Removing the traction weights and lowering the legs.
- Removing the bandages and extensions.
- Carrying out circulation checks every 15 minutes until the situation is reviewed.
- Keeping the limbs cool.

### 2. Skin breakdown

The following protocols will help to avoid skin breakdown:

a. The skin over the malleoli, the dorsum of the foot and behind the knee is routinely checked 4-hourly for signs of irritation and pressure. Bandages are adjusted and padding renewed as often as necessary, but at least daily.
b. The feet are oiled daily to keep the skin supple.
c. A sheepskin under the child helps to reduce the effects of pressure and friction (see Fig. 3.13). The skin overlying the occiput, scapulae and spine needs to be carefully inspected for signs of redness.

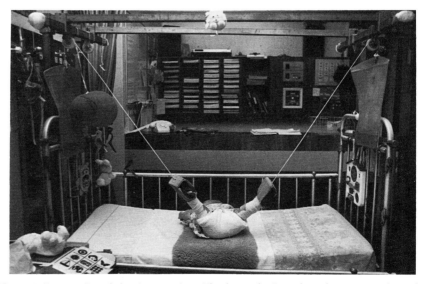

**Fig. 3.13** Progressive abduction traction. The buttocks just clear the mattress in order to obtain countertraction. A sheepskin under the child helps alleviate pressure and friction on the occiput scapulae and spine. The hips are abducted daily to the prescribed amount by moving the overhead bars and pulleys.

### 3. Indigestion

Feeds should be given slowly to prevent the accumulation of wind, which may result in distension and regurgitation. Smaller meals given more frequently may be preferable for the first 24 hours, or until the child becomes accustomed to the position.

### 4. Traction not proving effective

Follow-up X-rays will monitor the alignment of the fracture and the progress of healing.

**Variation 1**

Vertical lower limb traction (Bryant's traction, Gallows traction) can also be achieved without the use of pulleys and weights. The traction cords are simply tied to the overhead bar. The length of the cord is adjusted so that the buttocks just clear the mattress. The management is the same as for the traction above.

**Variation 2 (Progressive abduction traction)**

Progressive abduction traction (Modified Bryant's traction, Coronal traction, Divarication traction) is used in the management of congenital dislocation of the hip (Fig. 3.13). The child is positioned to lie across the cot. The hips are flexed to 90° and the legs are suspended vertically for 3–5 days. Then gradual abduction is commenced. A common regime is to move the pulleys apart by up to 5 cm (2 in) daily (Fig. 3.13). A potential problem added to those described for the traction above is painful stretching of the soft tissues, particularly the joint capsule, before the femoral head has been pulled down far enough to avoid impingement of the femoral head on the upper edge of the acetabulum. After each increase in abduction, the child is observed for signs of pain: restlessness and serious crying. If either of these occurs, the pulleys can be moved back to decrease the amount of abduction, and this should relieve the pain.

Follow-up X-rays are taken to determine the position of the femoral head in relation to the acetabulum. The observation of the circulation, the management of the skin, and feeding are the same as for the traction described above.

It is possible to move infants in this traction set-up onto the lap of a person seated beside the cot without disrupting the traction pull. Provided that the chair or stool beside the bed is the right height so that the lap is level with the mattress, the infant can be held for feeding and mothering.

## TWO-DIRECTIONAL LOWER LIMB TRACTION

HAMILTON RUSSELL TRACTION, RUSSELL TRACTION

This traction set-up (Fig. 3.14) described by R. Hamilton Russell in 1923 was devised by him to treat fractures of the femoral shaft. Nowadays, it is more commonly used for:

— conservative or temporary management of fractures of the femoral neck
— pre- and post-operative management of hip arthroplasty
— post-reduction management of hip dislocation
— femoral shaft fractures in children.

### Mechanics

Two forces are utilised to obtain a resultant pull in line with the long axis of the femur. The patient is recumbent with the hip and knee in slight flexion and the lower leg lying horizontally. The forces are applied as follows:

— A near-vertical pull is exerted on the leg via a sling cradling the knee.
— A horizontal pull is exerted simultaneously on the leg by means of below-knee skin extensions. This horizontal pull is nominally double that of the near-vertical pull because of the double-pulley system at the foot of the bed.

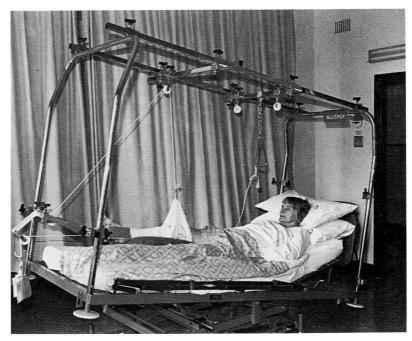

**Fig. 3.14** Hamilton Russell traction.

— The near-vertical pull and the horizontal pull acting together create a resultant pull in line with the long axis of the femur.
— Countertraction is obtained by elevating the foot of the bed (see Fig. 3.16).

**Requirements**

- Skin extensions complete with spreader to which a pulley is attached.
- A padded knee sling which is broad enough to prevent pressure behind the knee (Fig. 3.15).
- A soft pillow to support the leg. Two pillows may need to be used for a large patient.
- 1 bandage.
- 3 pulleys attached to the traction frame: one above the knee, or just distal to it, and two at the end of the bed, one above the other in line with the patient's foot (see Fig. 3.16).
- A single length of cord, approximately 8 metres (8½ yd) long.
- 2 blocks to elevate the end of the bed, if no tilt mechanism is available on the bed.
- 1 weight bag of the required weight, usually 2.7–3.6 kg (6–8 lb) for adults or 0.5–1.8 kg (1–4 lb) for children.
- Scissors.
- Tape measure.
- Skin preparation materials.
- Zinc oxide strapping 2.5 cm (1 in) wide.

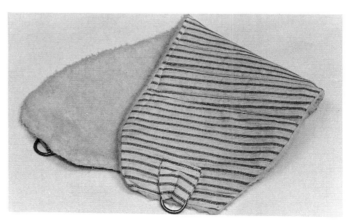

**Fig. 3.15** The knee sling should be reasonably broad and padded. The one illustrated is lined with sheepskin.

## Application

1. Assess and record the neurovascular status of the limb.
2. Apply the skin extensions to below the knee.
3. Place the sling under the knee and tie the traction cord to the eyelet ring or spreader bar of the sling.
4. Pass the traction cord in the following sequence (Fig. 3.16):

    a. up to pulley F1 above the leg
    b. out to pulley F2 at the end of the bed
    c. back to pulley S attached to the spreader
    d. out to pulley F3 at the end of the bed below pulley F2.

5. Tie the weight to the traction cord, allowing enough length to ensure that the weight hangs freely.

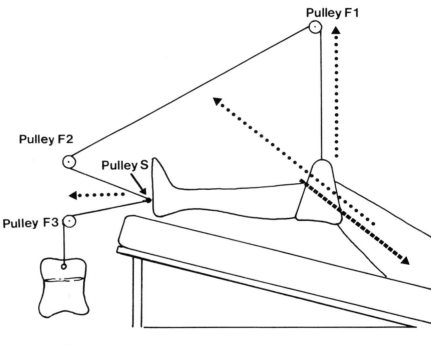

F = Frame
S = Spreader

**Fig. 3.16** Mechanics and application of Hamilton Russell traction. The pulleys are positioned and threaded in the sequence F1, F2, S, F3. The dotted lines denote the forces achieved by the vertical and horizontal traction pull. The resultant pull is consequently in line with the long axis of the femur. Countertraction (blocked line) is achieved by the patient's body weight when lying recumbent with the foot of the bed elevated.

6. Place a soft pillow under the leg to support the thigh and lower leg, leaving the heel free (Fig. 3.17).
7. Tape the cut ends of the traction cord.
8. Elevate the foot of the bed.
9. Check that:

   a. the pulley above the leg is just distal to the patella
   b. the sling is free from wrinkles
   c. the knee is flexed to provide an angle between the thigh and the mattress of approximately 20°
   d. the lower leg is parallel to the bed frame
   e. the heel is left free
   f. the foot of the bed is elevated approximately 15 cm (6 in).

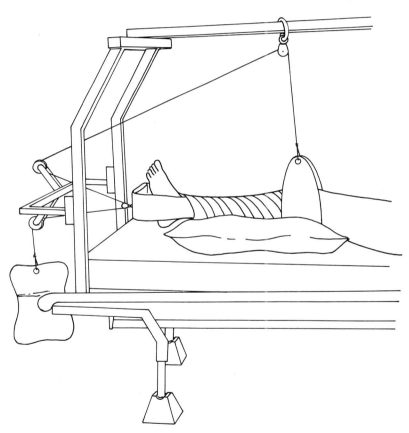

**Fig. 3.17** Hamilton Russell traction. The lower thigh, knee and lower leg are supported on the pillow leaving the heel clear.

**Potential problems**

1. Pressure in the politeal space

Inspect the skin under the sling 4-hourly and check that the sling is well padded. Ensure that the pillow is not too hard.

2. Pressure against the peroneal nerve over the head of the fibula

Check the padding. Use a spreader bar that is 5–7 cm (2–3 in) wider than the patient's knee to relieve the pressure of the sling. Monitor the patient's ability to dorsiflex the ankle.

3. Circulatory impairment due to tight bandages

Check the neurovascular status regularly. Investigate all complaints of numbness, tingling and pain.

4. Skin breakdown

— Check the skin extensions under the bandages for signs of irritation.
— Check that the heel is free from pressure.
— Teach the patient to lift up the trunk to ease pressure on the sacrum by grasping the trapeze bar and lifting the trunk while pushing up with the unaffected foot (see 'Aids to lifting and moving the patient', p. 8).
— Patients being treated for femoral shaft fractures are not turned but lifted for pressure care and placement of a bed pan. Use a mirror and torch to inspect the skin over the sacrum.
— All other patients can be turned. This is best accomplished as follows with the patient lying fairly flat in bed.

  a. Remove the pillow from under the leg and position it lengthwise between the legs, then
  b. logroll the patient approximately 45° to the side.

5. Traction not proving effective

Follow-up X-rays determine the progress of the treatment.

**Note**

a. The pulley above the knee determines the direction as well as the magnitude of the pull on the femur (see Fig. 3.16). Once the position is set it should not be altered without reference to the treating physician. An increase or decrease in the pulling force occurs, as does an alteration in the angle of the pull, if that pulley is moved, for example if the pulley is moved too far back towards the head of the bed, the upwards pull will be working somewhat against the longitudinal pull rather than combining with it, thus diminishing the pull.

b. If the pulleys on the foot end of the bed are placed too high, such that the lower leg is no longer lying horizontally and the foot is too elevated, some of the horizontal pull will be dissipated in counteracting the weight of the leg. The angle of the resultant pull will also be altered if the lower leg is not horizontal.

c. Countertraction is increased by further elevation of the foot of the bed.

**Variation (Modified Hamilton Russell traction, Split Russell traction)**

The upwards pull on the sling and the longitudinal pull on the leg are applied using separate cords and weights. The cord from the sling is carried from the pulley above the knee over another pulley at the head end of the bed. The cord from the spreader is passed over a single pulley attached to the frame at the foot end of the bed.

## STRAIGHT LEG FIXED SKIN TRACTION IN A THOMAS'S SPLINT

This traction set-up (Fig. 3.18) is commonly used in the management of femoral shaft fractures in older children. As a self-contained traction unit, it is used in the temporary management of similar fractures in adults who are to be transported.

### Mechanics

Traction and countertraction are exerted on the femur between two fixed points. The traction pull is exerted via skin extensions which are firmly tied to the end of the Thomas's splint (Fig. 3.19). The countertraction force is thus transmitted up the side bars of the splint to the ring which rests in the groin at the front and against the ischial tuberosity at the back (see Fig. 1.3 p. 5). Pulleys and weights are added to the system to provide suspension of the splint off the bed and to ease the pressure of the ring in the groin. The weights and pulleys do not contribute directly to the traction pull.

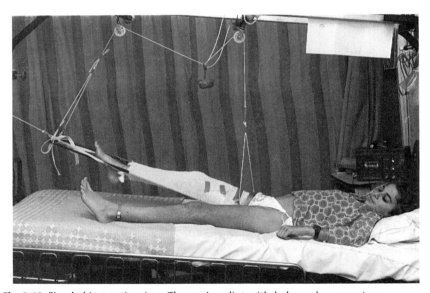

**Fig. 3.18** Fixed skin traction in a Thomas's splint with balanced suspension.

**Requirements**

- At least 2 assistants.
- Prepared skin extensions with lampwick ties (see Fig. 2.6 p. 22).
- An appropriately sized Thomas's splint.
- 3–5 calico or flannel slings to support the leg in the splint (Fig. 3.20).
- About 8 large safety pins to secure the slings.
- 1 cm ($\frac{1}{2}$ in) wide cotton tape to secure the proximal sling to the ring.
- 4 traction cords: one 3 m ($3\frac{1}{4}$ yd) long and three 1.5 m ($1\frac{2}{3}$ yd) long.
- Zinc oxide strapping 2.5 cm (1 in) wide.
- 2 weights of approximately 2.3 kg (5 lb) and 0.75 kg ($1\frac{1}{2}$ lb) respectively.

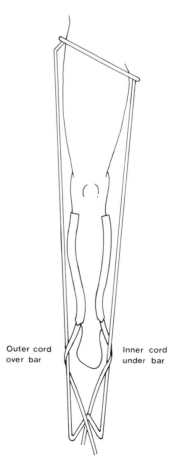

Outer cord
over bar

Inner cord
under bar

**Fig. 3.19** Fixed skin traction in a Thomas's splint. To minimise external rotation of the leg, the cord from the skin extension on the outside of the leg is passed first over then under the sidebar of the splint, and the inside cord is passed first under then over the bar before being tied securely to the end of the splint.

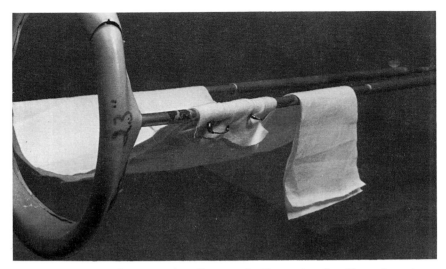

**Fig. 3.20** Positioning the supporting slings on the Thomas's splint. These flannel slings are pinned outside the outer side bar. They are placed loosely until the splint is threaded onto the leg, then they are tightened as needed.

- 2 bed blocks to elevate the foot of the bed if no tilt mechanism is available on the bed.
- 3 pulleys: 2 on the overhead bar and 1 on the frame at the foot end of the bed (see Fig. 3.22).
- Tape measure.
- Scissors.
- Skin preparation materials.

**Application**

1. Measuring and preparing the splint

**Note** Take the measurements from the uninjured leg to avoid causing the patient pain.

a. Length is estimated by measuring the distance from the adductor tendon in the groin to a point 25 cm (10 in) beyond the heel (Fig. 3.21).
b. Ring diameter is estimated by measuring obliquely from the adductor tendon in the groin, passing the tape under the gluteal fold just below the ischial tuberosity and over the greater trochanter (allow an additional 5 cm (2 in) to accommodate swelling). This oblique measurement corresponds to the angle that the ring makes with the inner bar. The diameter corresponds to the inside diameter of the ring.

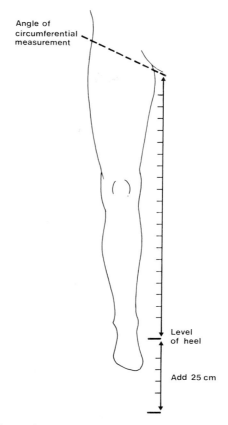

Angle of
circumferential
measurement

Level
of heel

Add 25 cm

**Fig. 3.21** Measuring for a Thomas's splint.

c. 3 to 5 slings are prepared from lengths of 15 cm (6 in) wide strong calico or flannel bandage. Each sling is doubled over the inner bar and secured to the lateral bar with safety pins (see Fig. 3.20). To prevent the slings from slipping down the bar, pin the proximal sling to a loop of cotton tape tied around the ring, and pin each sling to the one adjacent to it. The distal sling should end well above the heel to avoid pressure over the Achilles tendon.

d. Wool padding is placed on the slings to protect against pressure. A large pad of wool 20 cm (8 in) long by 5 cm (2 in) thick may be positioned under the thigh. This pad is placed by the treating physician according to the degree of knee flexion required and the amount of support needed to maintain the femur in satisfactory alignment. X-ray examination will confirm the position of the bone and indicate any adjustment needed.

2. Applying the skin extensions and splint

**Note** At least two assistants will be needed.

a. While manual traction is exerted on the leg and the knee and thigh are supported, apply the skin extensions as previously described (see Figs 3.2–3.8, pp. 27–30). The extensions should be applied only to the limb distal to the fracture site. Bandage over the extensions, leaving the patella exposed. Check and record the neurovascular status of the foot.
b. Thread the prepared Thomas's splint over the leg carefully while manual traction and support of the thigh are maintained. The ring of the splint should fit neatly in the groin and rest against the ischial tuberosity at the back. Adjust the tension of the slings to support the leg without causing undue pressure.
c. Fasten the skin extensions to the end of the Thomas's splint. In order to maintain neutral rotation of the limb, direct the lateral tie *over* the outer side bar and the medial tie *under* the inner side bar before tying them securely together at the end of the splint (see Fig. 3.19).

3 Suspending the splint

a. Attach a loop of cord to the side bars, at both the ring end and foot end of the splint.
b. Attach a length of cord to the loop on the ring end of the splint and pass it over the pulley directly above on the overhead bar. Attach the smaller weight to the cord and continue the cord over the pulley above the foot and down to the loop attached to the foot end of the splint (Fig. 3.22). To anchor the loop at the ring end of the splint, tie the cord to the ring with cotton tape (Fig. 3.23).
c. Tie a length of cord to the foot of the splint and pass it over the pulley on the crossbar and attach the 2.3 kg (5 lb) weight. This pull eases the pressure of the ring in the groin.
d. Loop a safety cord from the weight above the patient and tie it independently to the overhead bar (see Fig. 3.22).
e. Check that the back of the ring is the only part of the Thomas's splint to actually touch the bed.
f. Bandage the limb and the splint up to the groin, leaving the heel free and the patella exposed.
g. Tape the cut ends of the traction cord.
h. Elevate the foot of the bed.

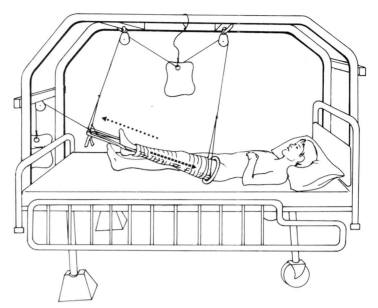

**Fig. 3.22** Suspending the Thomas's splint. Note the safety cord attached to the counterweight hanging above the patient.

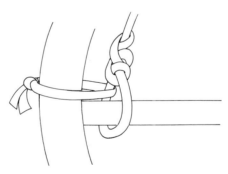

**Fig. 3.23** A piece of tape tied to the suspension cord prevents slippage along the sidebars.

**Potential problems**

1. Pressure in the groin

a. Routine skin care should include gently moving the skin underneath the ring to vary the pressure. Teach the patient to manage this if possible. Oiling the ring daily helps to reduce friction on the skin under the ring. It also keeps the ring covering soft and supple.

b. Check the amount of abduction. It may be necessary to increase the abduction slightly to ease the pressure. Sometimes this just means straightening the patient who has lost some abduction owing to tilting of the pelvis.

c. Have the patient lie down flat for longer periods to lessen the pressure.

### 2. Pressure at the back of the ring

Increasing the elevation of the foot of the splint may help to ease pressure here. Avoid padding the inside of the ring at the groin. This only results in increased pressure at the back by reducing the inside diameter of the ring.

### 3. Swelling

If gross swelling does occur, the ring may have to be cut off with bolt-cutters and a new splint applied.

### 4. Damage to skin, tendons and nerves from tight slings

Test the patient's ability to dorsiflex and plantarflex the foot and extend the toes. Check the position of the distal sling to ensure that the Achilles tendon is free from pressure. Adjust the slings under the calf and knee and renew the padding if necessary. Ensure that the area over the lateral aspect of the leg below the knee is well protected to prevent pressure on the common peroneal nerve, as this could result in foot drop.

### 5. Rotation of the splint

Adjust the suspension loops at the top and bottom ends of the splint to restore it to the neutral position. Tape the loops just below the knot to hold the corrected position (see Fig. 3.18). Leaving the patella exposed allows the rotation of the leg to be checked.

### 6. Loss of position of the fracture

Follow-up X-rays will reveal the problem and indicate the positional adjustments needed to maintain the correct alignment. Such correction is carried out by the treating physician. However, removal of the outer bandages daily will allow the general alignment of the limb to be noted. It should be observed from above and from the side to look for any change, for example sagging or deformity at the thigh. The ties from the extension to the end of the splint should remain taut. If they loosen, this should be reported to the treating physician or someone who is qualified to renew the traction pull by retying the ties to the splint.

### 7. Circulation impairment from tight wrapping bandages

Check the skin extensions for slipping and wrinkling, especially around the malleoli. Routine neurovascular assessments are continued throughout the traction treatment. Any deficit is reported at once and action is initiated immediately to restore the circulation. This may mean replacing the bandages, extensions or even the splint.

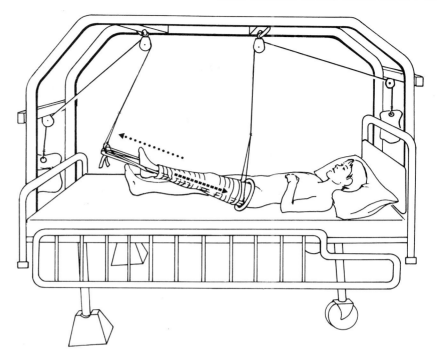

**Fig. 3.24** Alternative suspension of a Thomas's splint.

### Variation 1

An alternative means of suspending the Thomas's splint is accomplished using two separate sets of cords, pulleys and weights (Fig. 3.24). Clips can be used to attach the loops on the side bars to the main cords (Fig. 3.25).

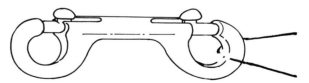

**Fig. 3.25** Clips provide an alternative means of joining the loops on the sidebars to the suspension cords.

### Variation 2 (Straight leg balanced traction — Yale method)

This is a balanced skin traction used in the management of femoral shaft fractures in children up to 10 years. Skin extensions incorporating a spreader are applied to the limb up to the fracture site. The limb is placed in a prepared Thomas's splint and elevated 40°–50°. The traction cord is tied to the spreader and carried over a pulley on the crossbar opposite the foot. The end of the Thomas's splint can be suspended as above or tied to a crossbar just below the pulley.

# 4 Skin traction to the upper limb

## EXTENDED SIDEARM FIXED TRACTION IN A THOMAS'S SPLINT

This set-up (Fig. 4.1) is used for the temporary management of displaced supracondylar fractures in children if vascular compromise occurs when manipulation and flexion of the elbow are attempted.

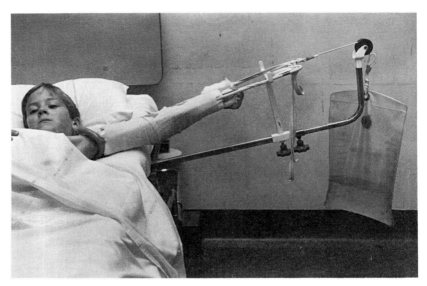

**Fig. 4.1** Extended sidearm fixed traction

### Mechanics

The child lies supine with the shoulder abducted and the elbow almost straight. Traction is exerted via skin extensions on the forearm which are tied to a Thomas's splint. The countertraction force is transmitted up the side bars of the splint to the ring (Fig. 4.2). A pulley and weight are used to maintain elevation and to ease the pressure of the ring against the axilla.

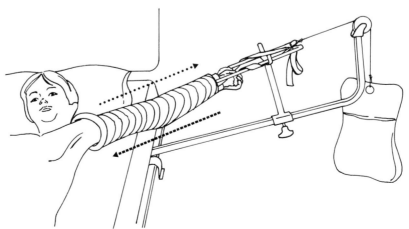

**Fig. 4.2** Elevating the arm in a Thomas's splint

### Requirements

- A sidearm frame with a pulley attached.
- A small Thomas's splint with slings attached (see Fig. 3.20 p. 46). Check the fit on the uninjured limb. The ring should fit the root of the arm snugly, and the end of the splint should extend 20 cm (8 in) beyond the hand (Fig. 4.2).
- Skin extensions cut to fit from just above the wrist to just below the elbow. They should be 5 cm (2 in) wide.
- Wool padding.
- 2 bandages.
- 1 length of traction cord 1.5 m (5 ft) long.
- 1 weight of 1.4 kg (3 lb).
- Scissors.
- Tape measure.
- Skin preparation materials.
- Zinc oxide strapping 2.5 cm (1 in) wide.

### Application

1. Clamp the sidearm frame securely to the bed frame in line with the long axis of the abducted arm.
2. Check the neurovascular status of the arm and record it as baseline information.
3. Pad the bony prominences around the elbow and wrist.
4. While the arm is being supported in extension and mild manual traction is being exerted, apply the skin extensions from just above the wrist to below the elbow on the medial and lateral aspects of the forearm.
5. Thread the prepared Thomas's splint over the arm.
6. Tie the lampwick ties on the extension tapes firmly to the end of the Thomas's splint (Fig. 4.3).

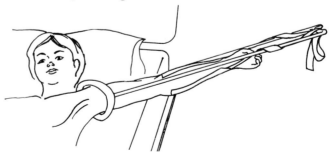

**Fig. 4.3** Applying the Thomas's splint. To minimize rotation the outer lampwick tie is passed under then over the sidebar; and the inner tie passes over then under the sidebar before being tied securely.

7. Bandage the arm over the extensions.
8. Attach the length of traction cord to the end of the splint, pass it over the pulley on the sidearm frame and attach the weight.
9. Tape the cut ends of the traction cords.
10. Bandage over the splint up to the ring (Fig. 4.4).

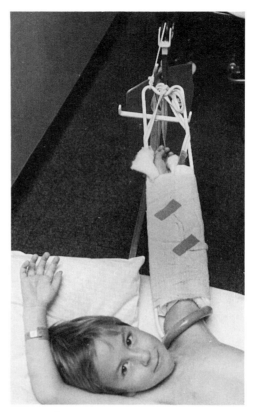

**Fig. 4.4** Overhead view of extended sidearm traction. Note that the Thomas's splint extends beyond the hand and that there is no pressure on the axilla.

### Potential problems

1. Neurovascular deficit

Hourly checks are essential for the first 24 hours to determine the status of the forearm. Undue pain plus any one of the following positive signs may indicate impending compartment syndrome:

- *Dulled sensation* — compare the affected limb with the uninjured limb.
- *Tense, tender forearm* — look and feel under the bandages.
- *Absent pulse* (but note that the presence of a pulse does *not* rule out ischaemia of the forearm).
- *Pain* on passive extension of the fingers.
- *Immediate steps must be taken to alert the treating physician if vascular compromise is suspected.*

2. Swelling of the hand

The bandages may be too tight or the hand may be too dependent. Encourage the child to flex and extend the fingers and wrist.

### 3. Pressure from the ring of the splint

Move the skin under the ring frequently to ease the pressure. Oil the ring daily to decrease friction. Tilt the child away slightly from the ring by placing a rolled towel under the mattress. Check the degree of abduction: it may need to be increased if it is less than 90°.

### 4. Pressure over bony prominences

Check the skin extensions for slipping and wrinkling. Renew padding over the wrist and around the elbow if needed.

### 5. Discomfort due to the enforced position

Inspect the skin over the shoulders, back, buttocks, heels and uninjured elbow for redness. Massage gently 2-hourly if necessary. Ensure that the child can reach easily any items that he or she needs.

## TWO-DIRECTIONAL UPPER LIMB TRACTION

DUNLOP TRACTION

This traction set-up (Fig. 4.5) is used to obtain gradual reduction of supracondylar and transcondylar fractures of the humerus in children.

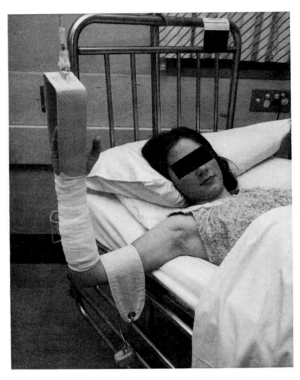

**Fig. 4.5** Two-directional upper limb traction. NB The radial pulse is difficult to palpate if the extensions cover the dorsal and ventral surfaces of the arm, as shown. See Figure 4.6 for preferable application.

## Mechanics

The shoulder is abducted 45° and the elbow is flexed to 45°. A lateral pull is exerted on the forearm via skin extensions, and a second force is directed downwards from the distal humerus by means of a weighted sling. These two forces, acting in different but not opposite directions, create a resultant force in line with the distal humerus (see Fig. 4.6 p. 60). Countertraction is achieved by means of the weight of the patient's body when the side of the bed or mattress is elevated.

## Requirements

- Skin extensions 5 cm (2 in) wide, with spreader included.
- A padded sling.
- 2 weights, the amount depending on the weight of the child. Approximately 1 kg (2.2 lb) for the forearm weight and 0.5 kg (1 lb) for the sling weight is generally sufficient initially.
- 1 length of traction cord of about 2 m ($2\frac{1}{4}$ yd).
- 1 bandage.
- Wool padding.
- 2 blocks or a rolled blanket to elevate the side of the bed or mattress.
- A sideframe with pulley attached, or a projecting overhead crossbar with pulley attached.
- Scissors.
- Tape measure.
- Skin preparation materials.
- Zinc oxide strapping 2.5 cm (1 in) wide.

## Application

1. Record the neurovascular status of the limb.
2. Position the child supine with the shoulder abducted approximately 45° and the upper arm clear of the bed.
3. Pad the bony prominences around the wrist and elbow with wool.
4. Apply the skin extensions over the medial and lateral aspects of the forearm. The extensions end just below the elbow, and the spreader extends at least 10 cm (4 in) beyond the hand.
5. Bandage over the extensions.

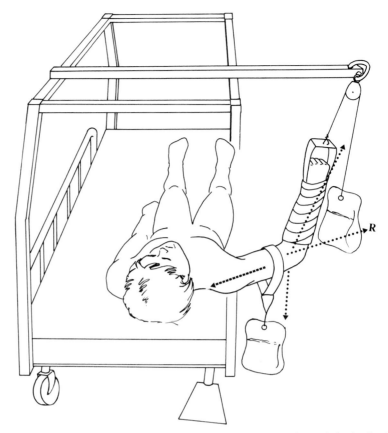

**Fig. 4.6** Applying Dunlop traction. Note that the upper arm is free of the bed. The two traction forces produce a resultant pull (R) in line with the distal humerus. Counter traction is achieved by elevating the bed (or mattress) on the affected side.

6. Tie the length of cord to the spreader and pass it over the pulley, maintaining the elbow at approximately 45° of flexion (Fig. 4.6).
7. Place the padded sling over the distal humerus and hang the second weight from it.
8. Tape the cut ends of the traction cord.
9. Elevate the side of the bed with blocks, or pad the mattress on the affected side with the rolled blanket.
10. Check that:

    a. the elbow is flexed to approximately 45°.
    b. the shoulder is abducted to approximately 45°.
    c. the upper arm is clear of the bed.
    d. the weight hanging from the sling is hanging freely.

**Potential problems**

1. Neurovascular deficit

The circulation must be checked hourly for the first 12 to 24 hours, then 2- to 4-hourly for the remainder of the time the traction is being exerted. The signs to watch for are the same as those listed in 'Extended Sidearm traction' described on page 56.

2. Swelling at the elbow due to a tight bandage

Make sure the bandage is not too tightly wrapped.

3. Swelling of the hand and fingers

Encourage movement of the fingers by the patient. Check that the extension spreader is wide enough and far enough away from the hand to permit free movement.

4. Skin breakdown due to extensions and bandages

Check under the bandages for signs of irritation and pressure. Increase or replace the padding as necessary.

## OVERHEAD FLEXED ARM TRACTION

OVERHEAD 90–90 TRACTION

This traction set-up (Fig. 4.7) is used when relatively light traction is needed to immobilise and maintain the reduction of the proximal humerus and shoulder.

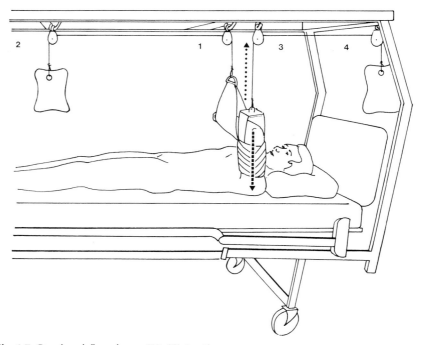

**Fig. 4.7** Overhead flexed arm (90–90) traction.

### Mechanics

The patient lies flat in bed with the elbow and shoulder flexed to 90°. Vertical traction is exerted via skin extensions on the humerus. The forearm is supported in a sling suspended above the patient's chest. Because a vertical traction pull is used, countertraction is achieved by means of the weight of the patient's arm.

### Requirements

- A set of 5 cm (2 in) wide skin extensions with spreader attached. Measure from below the fracture site to 6 cm (2½ in) beyond the point of the elbow.
- Wool padding.
- 1 bandage.
- 1 padded sling.

- 4 pulleys: 2 placed on the crossbar directly above the elbow and the forearm, and 2 placed in line with these pulleys towards the end(s) of the bed.
- Traction cord 6–7 m (20–25 ft) long cut into two equal lengths.
- 2 weights: up to 2.7 kg (6 lb) for the traction on the humerus, and approximately 1–1.5 kg (2–3 lb) to suspend the forearm, depending on the size and weight of the patient.
- Scissors.
- Tape measure.
- Skin preparation materials.
- Zinc oxide strapping 2.5 cm (1 in) wide.

## Application

1. Position the patient flat with one pillow under the head.
2. Tie one length of cord to the spreader on the extensions and the other to the sling.
3. Record the neurovascular status of the limb.
4. While the arm is being supported in 90° of flexion at both the shoulder and the elbow, slip the sling over the forearm. Pass the cord from the sling over pulleys 1 and 2 and attach the smaller weight.
5. Pad the elbow and wrist with wool.
6. Apply the skin extensions to the upper arm, placing them parallel on the medial and lateral aspects of the arm. They should begin distal to the fracture site and allow a 6 cm (2½ in) gap between the arm and the spreader.
7. Wrap the bandage over the extensions at half stretch.
8. Pass the cord from the spreader over pulleys 3 and 4 and attach the heavier weight.
9. Tape the cut ends of the traction cord.
10. Check that the shoulder and elbow are flexed to 90°.

## Potential problems

1. Circulatory impairment

Monitor the neurovascular status of the limb (see pp. 14–16) and check the tightness of the bandages.

2. Swelling of the hand

Make sure the wrist and forearm are fully supported by the sling and not allowed to become dependent. Encourage active movement of the fingers and hand by the patient.

3. Swelling at the elbow and shoulder

Check that the wrapping bandage is not too tight and adjust if necessary.

4. Skin breakdown

— Check the skin extension edges for signs of slipping and irritation.
— Check that padding is sufficient around the bony prominences at the elbow and wrist. Ensure that the distal edge of the bandage is not digging into the front of the elbow.
— Check the forearm inside the sling.
— Inspect the skin over the heels, buttocks and sacrum regularly for signs of pressure. Encourage the patient to lift the buttocks off the bed to relieve pressure whilst keeping the shoulders against the mattress. To attend to the skin under the shoulders, depress the mattress firmly and slide the hand in under the scapulae.

**Variation (90–90 Sidearm traction)**

2 sets of skin extensions are used: 1 set on the upper arm, and 1 set on the forearm. The patient is supine with the shoulder abducted to 90°. Lateral traction is exerted in a straight line with the humerus. The elbow is flexed to 90° and suspended vertically.

# 5 Circumferential and sling traction to the spine and pelvis

Circumferential skin traction to the cervical spine
  Halter traction, Glisson sling traction
    Mechanics
    Requirements
    Application
    Potential problems
    Variation
Intermittent longitudinal back traction
  Cotrel's traction
    Mechanics
    Requirements
    Application
    Potential problems
Circumferential pelvic belt traction
  Pelvic harness traction
    Mechanics
    Requirements
    Application
    Potential problems
    Variation 1
    Variation 2
Intermittent dynamic 90–90 back traction
    Mechanics
    Requirements
    Application
Balanced vertical pelvic traction
  Pelvic sling traction, pelvic suspension traction
    Mechanics
    Requirements
    Application
    Potential problems

## CIRCUMFERENTIAL SKIN TRACTION TO THE CERVICAL SPINE

## HALTER TRACTION, GLISSON SLING TRACTION

In this balanced skin traction (Fig. 5.1), a traction pull is exerted on the cervical spine by means of a halter which encircles the head at the occiput and the chin. It is most often used in the management of neck pain due to degenerative changes in the cervical spine causing muscle spasm and nerve impingement. This traction is usually prescribed for intermittent use as continuous use is not well tolerated, due to pressure on the chin and difficulties with eating. Careful note is made of any pertinent change in the patient's symptoms when traction is released. If the patient is allowed out of bed and is on analgesic or muscle relaxing drugs, he or she must be supervised because of the risk of falls due to the medication.

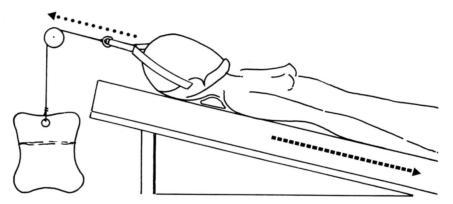

**Fig. 5.1** Circumferential skin traction to the cervical spine.

### Mechanics

The patient lies flat in bed with a small, soft neck support in place. Traction is exerted in a straight line by means of a weight attached by a cord to a spreader on the halter. Countertraction is provided by the patient's weight when the head end of the bed is elevated. Usually between 1.4–2.3 kg (3–5 lb) weight traction is sufficient. The maximum weight 2.3 kg (5 lb) is never exceeded. If a larger traction pull is required, skeletal traction is used.

### Requirements

- Head halter.
- Spreader bar.
- Traction cord 1.5 m (5 ft) long.
- Pulley or pulleys according to the type of frame in use.
- Soft neck support.
- Weight.
- Bed blocks to elevate the head of the bed, if needed.

### Application

1. Position the patient flat with a neck support in position.
2. Position the pulley on the traction frame in line with the top of the patient's head.
3. Fit the halter on the patient's head so that the front piece is centred over the chin and the back piece is over the occiput. Check that the side straps are not pressing on the ears.
4. Tie one end of the traction cord to the spreader and pass the cord over the pulley.
5. Hook the spreader bar onto the head halter straps.
6. Attach the weight to the free end of the traction cord beyond the pulley, allowing enough length to let the weight hang freely.
7. Elevate the head end of the bed.

### Potential problems

1. Pressure and irritation under the halter

a. Inspect the skin under the chin piece and over the occiput for signs of pressure.
b. Protect the chin piece from spilt liquids when the patient drinks by tucking a protective cloth over the chin piece and using angled straws in drinking glasses that are only half full.
c. If the ears are rubbed by the side straps, use a wider spreader or two separate pulleys placed far enough apart to leave the ears free.
d. Male patients may find that beard stubble is irritating under the chin piece and will need to shave each day. Bearded patients vary in their tolerance to chin pressure. Some might prefer to shave the beard.

2. Ineffective traction

a. Uneven pull. Check that the spreader is level and that the halter is centred on the head.
b. If intermittent traction is prescribed, plan the patient's daily regime to ensure that the requisite time is spent in traction. Provide prism glasses, angled mirrors and reading stands to increase the patient's tolerance to the traction periods. These aids will allow the patient to read or write comfortably and maintain eye contact with others.
c. If the spreader keeps touching the bed frame, either increase the countertraction by elevating the head of the bed still further or, in the case of a very tall patient, remove the bed end-board and add a mattress extension.

d. If the patient is allowed up, check after each resumption of the traction that the alignment is correct. It is worthwhile teaching the patient how to get up without putting strain on the neck. This is done by turning onto the side and pushing up into a sitting position using the arms.

**Variation**

If positional adjustments are available on the bed, the patient may be able to have the head and shoulders raised higher while the traction pull is maintained in line with the neck.

## INTERMITTENT LONGITUDINAL BACK TRACTION

### COTREL'S TRACTION

This dynamic traction set-up (Fig. 5.2) is used in some centres as an adjunct to pre-operative bracing in the management of scoliosis. The traction apparatus consists of a head halter, pelvic belt, and foot pieces (Fig. 5.2A). The patient initiates the traction pull. The traction treatment is usually given two or three times daily and converted into a static traction at night for sleeping.

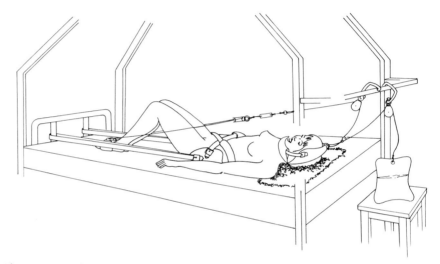

**Fig. 5.2A** Cotrel's traction apparatus in the relaxed position.

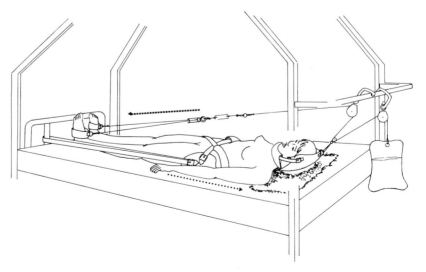

**Fig. 5.2B** Cotrel's traction. The patient exerts traction on the spine by extending the legs and pushing down on the foot pieces.

### Mechanics

A longitudinal pull is exerted on the spine by means of a traction weight attached to the head halter, and foot pieces attached to the patient's feet. Countertraction is supplied by a pelvic belt which stabilises the pelvis and is fixed by two long sidestraps to the frame at the end of the bed. The patient initiates the traction force by extending the legs, thus pushing the foot pieces against the pull of the head halter (Fig. 5.2B). No elevation of the bed is necessary.

### Requirements

- Cotrel's traction apparatus.
- Two pulleys.
- Weight — usually 2.3–3.2 kg (5–7 lb) is used initially. This can be gradually increased.
- A clip or ring connection.
- A traction hook or spreader.
- Traction cord approximately 3–4 m (10 ft) long.
- Soft neck support.

### Application

1. Position the two pulleys on the frame at the head of the bed.
2. With the patient lying flat apply the pelvic band so that its upper border encircles the hips, not the waist.
3. Adjust the side straps on the pelvic belt so that each strap can be fixed to the bed frame.
4. Place the foot pieces on the patient and adjust the attached loop so that it comes up to the patient's pelvis.
5. Fit the head halter on the patient ensuring that it is evenly centred over the chin.
6. Place the neck support in position.
7. Attach a pulley to the halter.
8. Tie the traction cord to the foot piece loop and pass it over the pulleys as follows:

   — over the top pulley
   — back to the halter pulley
   — out to the bottom pulley.

9. Attach the weight allowing enough length of traction cord to allow the weight to hang freely.

### Potential problems

Temporomandibular pain

With prolonged use, there may be some pain in the temporomandibular joints. This may be relieved by the use of a bite block or by reducing the weight and frequency of the traction.

**Conversion to static traction**

Static traction can be maintained at night by removing the foot pieces and passing the cord from the head halter over a single pulley.

## CIRCUMFERENTIAL PELVIC BELT TRACTION

### PELVIC HARNESS TRACTION

This traction set-up (Fig. 5.3) is used in the management of low back pain due to a prolapsed intervertebral disc. The belt is made of canvas in a variety of sizes, with adjustable long sidestraps. A disposable type is available with Velcro fasteners which can be cut to fit the patient.

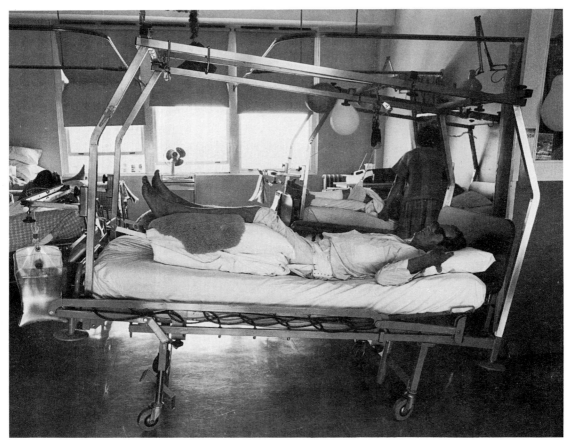

**Fig. 5.3** Circumferential pelvic belt traction. The head board is raised slightly to keep the head and shoulders level with the trunk. A sheepskin is under the legs and the heels making them free of pressure. (Photograph courtesy Department of Illustrations, Concord Hospital, Sydney, New South Wales.)

### Mechanics

Traction is exerted on the pelvis via a weight attached to the side straps of the belt. Countertraction is provided by the patient's weight when the foot of the bed is elevated. The patient is positioned to lie with the legs either extended or with the hips and knees well flexed and supported on pillows — the so-called 'astronaut position'.

### Requirements

- An appropriately-sized pelvic belt. It should fit snugly around the iliac crests proximally and over the trochanters distally.
- Spreader bar.
- Pulley.
- Traction cord, approximately 2 m (6 ft) long.
- Pillows or foam wedges to support the legs.
- Weight — generally 4.5 kg (10 lb) is sufficient to begin with; the weight may be gradually increased.
- Blocks to elevate the foot of the bed.

### Application

1. Position the pulley on the frame at the foot of the bed in line with the patient's spine.
2. Secure the pelvic belt around the patient's hips.
3. Adjust the length of the side straps so that they extend 25 cm (10 in) beyond the feet.
4. Position the pillows or foam blocks under the legs.
5. Tie the traction cord to the spreader and hook the spreader to the side straps.
6. Pass the cord from the spreader over the pulley and attach the weight.
7. Elevate the foot end of the bed.
8. Raise the head board slightly to keep the patient's head and shoulders level with the trunk (Fig. 5.4).

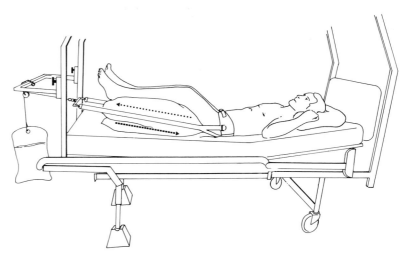

**Fig. 5.4** Pelvic belt traction. The patient is in the 'astronaut' position with knees and hips well flexed.

## Potential problems

### 1. Discomfort over the iliac crests and skin irritation

Check that the belt is not loose and slipping down. Thin patients may need extra padding over the bony prominences. Routine skin care includes inspection of the skin over iliac crests and trochanters. Wearing the belt next to the skin achieves a better grip. However, if the patient is allowed up, it is usually put on over the night clothes. In this case, cotton clothing is preferable.

### 2. Problems with elimination

If the patient is confined to bed, a fracture bed pan can be positioned by easing the pillows down and folding the distal end of the pelvic belt back. The lower front fastenings of the belt may need to be loosened slightly. If the patient's condition allows, he or she may use the trapeze to lift up while the pan is placed in position. Otherwise, the patient can be logrolled to one side with a pillow between the legs and rolled back onto the pan.

## Variation 1

Instead of a spreader bar, two separate cords are attached to the side straps and directed over pulleys to two weights (Fig. 5.5). The weight must be equal on each side.

## Variation 2

The patient can be positioned without pillows under the legs (Fig. 5.5). The heels are prone to pressure in this position. Care must be taken to cover the patient's legs adequately and a bed cradle may be required to keep the bed clothes off the side straps or cords.

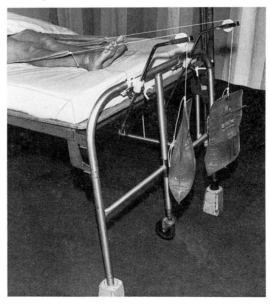

**Fig. 5.5** Pelvic belt traction — Variations 1 and 2.

## INTERMITTENT DYNAMIC 90–90 BACK TRACTION

This traction (Fig. 5.6) is used in the management of recurrent attacks of acute backache due to degenerative changes in the lumbar spine. The traction apparatus is portable, consisting of a pelvic belt with a tail piece and a frame with a pulley device attached. A foam wedge and block support the patient in a recumbent position with the knees and hips flexed to 90°. The traction is operated by the patient and is used intermittently during the day.

### Mechanics

Traction is exerted by the patient pulling on the hand grip with sufficient force to lift the buttocks off the bed, thus tilting the pelvis and overcoming lumbar lordosis.

### Requirements

- Frame (includes pulley device and hand grip).
- Pelvic belt with tail piece.
- Traction cord 1.5 m (5 ft) long.
- Shoulder and leg supports.
- Pillow.

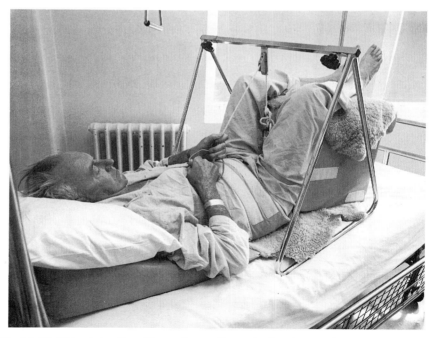

**Fig. 5.6** 90–90 back traction. The patient pulls on the handgrip to lift the buttocks up off the bed. (Photograph courtesy Department of Illustrations, Concord Hospital, Sydney, New South Wales.)

**Application**

1. Place the wedge and pillow under the patient's head and shoulders.
2. Position the opened pelvic belt under the patient's pelvis with the V-shaped tail piece pointing towards the foot of the bed.
3. Tie the traction cord to the D ring on the tail piece.
4. Wrap the belt around the patient's hips and fasten the Velcro straps. It should fit snugly but not be uncomfortably tight. Bring the tail piece up between the patient's legs.
5. Position the portable frame over the patient so that the pulley is in line with the D ring on the tail piece.
6. Pass the cord through the pulley device and attach it to the hand grip.
7. Place the foam block under the patient's legs to maintain the hips and knees in 90° of flexion.
8. Adjust the length of the cord, if necessary, to permit the patient to pull effectively in order to lift the buttocks off the bed.

## BALANCED VERTICAL PELVIC TRACTION

PELVIC SLING TRACTION, PELVIC SUSPENSION TRACTION

This type of traction (Fig. 5.7) is used in the management of minimally displaced fractures of the pelvic rim when a mild compressive force is required. It is combined with skeletal lower limb traction to the affected side when there is upwards displacement of one side of the pelvis.

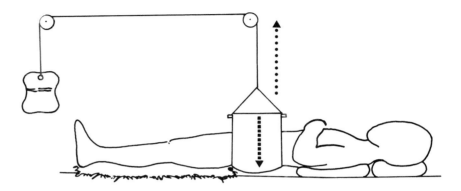

**Fig. 5.7** Balanced vertical pelvic traction.

### Mechanics

A vertical traction pull with enough weight to suspend the patient's pelvis just clear of the mattress is exerted by means of a pelvic sling. Countertraction is provided by the patient's body weight. A mild compressive force is exerted on the iliac bones by the sides of the sling. The amount of compression can be increased by pulling the sides of the sling towards the midline. This is accomplished by using an adjustable pelvic sling spreader, or by crossing the suspension cords above the patient as shown in Figure 5.8. The amount of weight required depends on the weight of the patient and the amount of compression needed. Commonly, 4.5 kg (10 lb) is used initially; this is gradually increased if indicated by X-ray evaluation.

### Requirements

- Pelvic sling with wooden rods threaded through each hem (Fig. 5.9).
- Two traction cords, each 4.5 m (15 ft) long.
- Pelvic sling spreader, or two cord loops.
- 2 or 4 pulleys, depending on the set-up used (Figs 5.7 and 5.8).
- 2 weights.
- 2 small pillows to support the head and shoulders.

**Application**

1. Position the pulleys on the overhead bar to achieve a vertical pull from the sling (Fig. 5.7). If the suspension cords are to be crossed over, position the pulleys as shown in Figure 5.8.
2. Position the sling under the patient so that it cradles the area from the posterior iliac crests to the gluteal fold.
3. Attach a loop of cord to each rod in the hem of the sling or position the spreader.
4. Tie the traction suspension cords to each loop, or to the spreader, and pass them over the pulleys.
5. Attach the weights.
6. Place the head and shoulder pillows so that the patient's trunk is level.

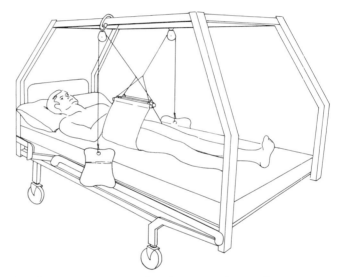

**Fig. 5.8** Pelvic sling traction. By crossing the suspension cords, a greater compressive force is achieved.

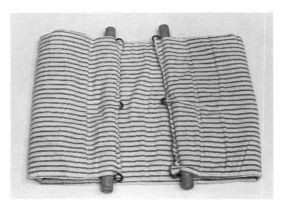

**Fig. 5.9** Pelvic sling. This consists of two layers of heavy cotton material with an inner foam layer to provide padding. A wooden rod is threaded through each hem. Metal rings are screwed into the rods for traction cord attachment.

**Potential problems**

1. Venous stasis in the legs

The risk of deep venous thrombosis can be reduced by ensuring that no pillows are placed under the knees. A sheepskin placed under the whole length of the legs will promote comfort and avoid prolonged flexion of the knees. Anti-embolism stockings may be prescribed. Hourly ankle and leg exercises are essential; the use of a bed cradle over the lower legs will facilitate the leg exercises.

2. Problems with elimination, hygiene and skin care

If only a mild degree of compression is exerted, the sling can be gently eased up towards the waist for the positioning of the fracture bed pan. Female patients may be able to use a female urinal or may have an indwelling catheter. Washing of the perineum and buttocks and massage of the skin over the sacrum can be carried out while the sling is eased back. The lower end of the sling needs to be protected from soiling and wetting when the pan is used. If the sling does become wet or soiled, it should be changed. A torch and mirror is useful to inspect the skin over the sacrum and buttocks. The skin in the lumbar region and iliac crests can be massaged by easing a hand under the upper edge of the sling.

These procedures are much more difficult when the compression force is greater. The decision may be made by the treating physician to permit temporary reduction of the compression force for the positioning of the fracture bed pan and skin care.

# 6 Skeletal traction

## METHODS OF APPLYING SKELETAL TRACTION TO THE UPPER AND LOWER LIMBS

Skeletel traction is applied directly to bone by means of pins, wires or traction screws. It is used when large traction forces are needed to overcome the powerful pull of muscles in the management of fractures of the lower limbs, pelvis and the cervical spine. Sufficient force can be transmitted directly to bone to obtain the reduction of the fracture and to maintain the position and stability of the fracture in good alignment. Weights of up to 18 kg (40 lb) can be used, depending on the fracture and the density of the bone at the insertion site. Lighter weights with skeletal traction may be used in instances when skin traction is contraindicated.

The application of skeletal traction is a surgical procedure performed under full aseptic conditions and requiring the informed consent of the patient. A hand drill is used to insert the pin under general or local anaesthesia. The neurovascular status of the affected part should be recorded prior to insertion of the pin.

In long bones, stainless steel pins or wires are connected to special stirrups or traction bows, or special swivels, which direct the traction cord to the weight. A variety of devices is available and usually some type of frame or splint is used to support and suspend the limb.

1. *Kirschner wires* have the smallest diameter, ranging from 0.07–1.6 mm (0.028–0.62 in). These wires can only be used with a *Kirschner traction bow* or *strainer*, which is designed to provide the slender wire with rigidity by exerting on it a longitudinal tension force.
2. *Steinmann pins* are unthreaded stainless steel pins of varying lengths and diameters and have either a diamond shaped or trocar point.
3. *Denham pins* have a raised threaded section which engages in the cortex of the bone. This allows greater purchase on the bone reducing the risk of movement, particularly lateral sliding of the pin in cancellous or osteoporotic bone. This pin also comes in a range of diameters and lengths, with a choice of either a trocar or diamond point. The protruding ends of the pins or wire should be capped to prevent inadvertent injury to the patient or staff.
4. The *Böhler stirrup* is the traction bow that is attached to the skeletal pin ends to carry the traction cord to the weight (Fig. 6.1). Another way of attaching the traction cord to the skeletal pins is by means of two low friction swivels.

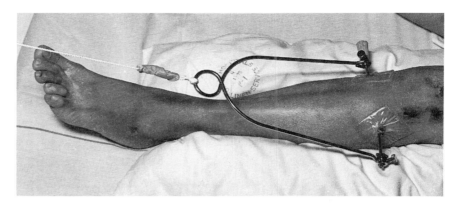

**Fig. 6.1** Skeletal traction at the upper tibial site. A Böhler stirrup clamped onto a Steinmann or Denham pin carries the traction cord to the weight. Note the cork capping the sharp point on the pin. The pin insertion sites are covered by an occlusive dressing.

5. *Simonis swivels*, made of thermoplastic and stainless steel, are particularly useful when skeletal traction without any external splintage or support is used. Such traction set-ups are designed to allow maximum movement of the joints without interfering with the traction pull. Examples are Perkins traction for femoral shaft fractures and calcaneal traction for tibial fractures (Fig. 6.2).

6. Pelvic traction screws (*Green's screw, Zimmer screw*) are inserted into the proximal femur in the management of displaced acetabular fractures. A smaller screw eye is used at the olecranon site.

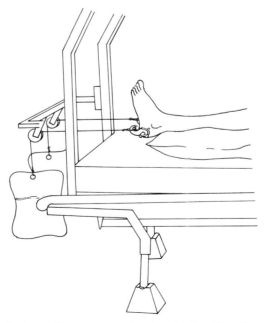

**Fig. 6.2** Skeletal traction at the calcaneal site. Low friction Simonis swivels are used to carry the traction cords from the skeletal pin to the weights. The swivels rotate smoothly around the pin preventing movement of the pin itself.

COMMON SITES OF INSERTION OF SKELETAL TRACTION
DEVICES

### Upper limb

*The olecranon site* is used in the management of supra-condylar and
comminuted fractures of the distal humerus and in unstable humeral
shaft fractures.

Kirschner wire is inserted from the medial side at right angles to
the longitudinal axis of the ulna, approximately 3 cm (1.25 in) distal
to the tip of the olecranon. Traction weight of 1.3–1.8 kg (3–4 lb) is
generally sufficient. The direction of the traction pull and the suspension of the forearm is determined by the degree of angulation and
rotation at the fracture site needing correction. The traction pull may
be:

a. Vertical, with the forearm across the chest as in overhead 90–90
   skin traction (see Fig. 4.7).
b. Horizontal, with the shoulder abducted to 45° and the pull
   directed laterally to a pulley on the side frame. The forearm is
   supported by means of skin extensions.
c. Almost horizontal, with the shoulder slightly abducted (just
   enough to keep the pin end from touching the chest) and the traction pull directed over a pulley at the foot end of the bed. The
   forearm is suspended by slings or skin extensions in a vertical
   position.

*The metacarpal site* is used in the management of comminuted fractures of the radius and ulna and sometimes in combination with
olecranon traction when there is a fracture of the humerus on the
same limb.

A Kirschner wire is passed through the second and third metacar-
pals at right angles to the long axis of the radius. The traction pull
is directed vertically over a pulley on the overhead bar. Countertraction is provided by the weight of the arm when the elbow is clear of
the bed. Additional countertraction can be obtained by the use of a
weighted sling over the upper arm as used in Dunlop skin traction
(Figs. 4.5 and 4.6).

Once satisfactory alignment of the fracture is evident, the Kirschner
wire is incorporated in an above-elbow cast. The patient is encouraged to move the fingers through as wide a range as possible as a
potential problem of this type of traction is stiffness of the fingers due
to fibrosis of the interosseus muscles.

### Lower limb

*Lateral upper femur.* This site is used in the management of acetabular fractures of the pelvis. It is also used simultaneously with
longitudinal traction on the femur for the management of central fracture dislocations of the hip.

A pelvic traction screw is inserted through a small longitudinal
incision just below the prominence on the trochanter. The traction

pull is directed to a pulley on the side frame in line with the long axis of the femoral neck. Between 4.5 kg–9 kg (10–20 lb) is usually enough weight. Countertraction is obtained by raising the side of the bed so that the patient is tilted away from the traction pull (Fig. 6.3). If the lateral femoral traction is combined with longitudinal traction, the bed will need to be tilted in two planes to achieve countertraction (Fig. 6.4).

The patient is encouraged to perform active hip and knee movements and to tilt himself or herself off the mattress toward the traction force to ease the pressure on the sacral area. This manoeuvre is accomplished by grasping the trapeze bar while pushing down with the unaffected foot. A long-handled mirror and a torch will help in

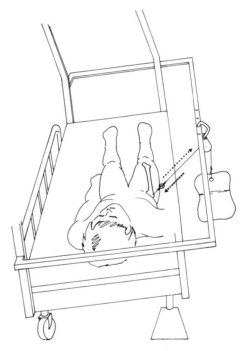

**Fig. 6.3** Skeletal traction at the lateral upper femoral site. A pelvic traction screw directs the traction cord to the weight on a side frame. Countertraction is maintained by tilting the bed on blocks on the affected side.

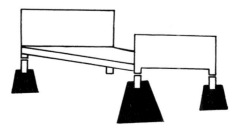

**Fig. 6.4** Placement of bed blocks to tilt the bed in two planes. This arrangement is necessary when longitudinal traction is used simultaneously with lateral upper femoral traction to ensure countertraction exists for each traction pull.

the inspection of vulnerable pressure sites. Pin site breakdown is a potential problem due in part to the amount of soft tissue impaled by the traction screw. Careful inspection of the pin site, particularly just underneath the screw on the lateral thigh, is needed to watch for early signs of increased tissue pressure.

*The distal femoral site* is used in the management of some pelvic fractures and following resection of the femoral head. A Steinmann or Denham pin is inserted from the medial side approximately 2.5 cm (1 in) inferior to the adductor tubercle.

*The proximal tibial site* is used in the management of femoral fractures. The pin is inserted from the lateral side to avoid damage to the common peroneal nerve.

*The distal tibial site* is sometimes utilised to treat tibial plateau fractures and in the short-term management of tibial shaft fractures. The pin is inserted parallel to the ankle joint approximately 3 cm ($1\frac{1}{4}$ in) above the malleolus. The traction bow or stirrup must be large enough to extend clear of the patient's foot.

*The calcaneal site* (see Fig. 6.2) is used in the temporary management of lower leg fractures. The insertion site is either 2.5 cm (1 in) inferior and posterior to the lateral malleolus or 4.5 cm ($1\frac{3}{4}$ in) inferior and 3.8cm ($1\frac{1}{2}$ in) posterior to the medial malleolus. The lower leg is elevated on a pillow or supported on a Böhler-Braun frame.

## METHODS OF SUSPENDING THE LOWER LIMB IN SKELETAL TRACTION

By means of balanced suspension the limb is elevated and supported, allowing the patient freedom to move and exercise without disrupting the mechanics of the traction system. A variety of splints are used to achieve balanced suspension.

### 1. Balanced suspension in a Thomas's splint

For the measurements and preparation of the Thomas's splint see pages 46–47. The splint is modified by the addition of a knee flexion piece (Pearson attachment) to allow flexion of the knee. It is important that the knee flexion piece hinges exactly at the level of the axis of movement of the knee. A landmark on the leg corresponding to this point is the adductor tubercle on the femur. The degree of flexion is controlled by the length of the cords joining the distal ends of the knee piece and the Thomas's splint.

The splint is suspended using cords, weights and pulleys as shown in Figure 6.5. The amount of weight required to suspend the splint depends on the weight of the leg and the splint and the amount of friction inherent in the system. The only part of the splint which remains in contact with the bed is the back of the padded ring. When

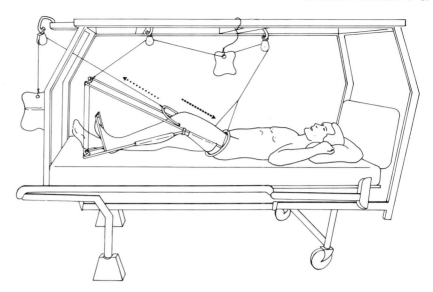

**Fig. 6.5** Skeletal traction in balanced suspension in a Thomas's splint. Countertraction is achieved by elevating the foot of the bed.

the patient lifts up using the trapeze bar and the unaffected foot, the whole of the splint and limb move as a single unit with the patient's trunk. Countertraction to the skeletal traction pull is achieved by elevating the foot of the bed.

The addition of a foot piece (Fig. 6.6) to the knee flexion piece level with the sole of the foot provides support. This support combined with active dorsiflexion exercises helps to prevent equinus deformity of the ankle due to weakness of the muscles. The foot piece frame is covered by a sling of elastic material such as elastic tubular bandage. The patient is encouraged to actively dorsiflex and plantar flex the foot throughout the day and the foot is supported in a good position during sleep.

Routine skin care is aimed at preventing pressure and friction from the ring of the splint and the supporting slings as previously described on page 49.

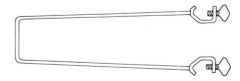

**Fig. 6.6** A foot piece frame covered by elastic tubular bandage provides support for the foot and resistive exercises for the ankle. It is clamped securely to the lower end of the knee piece as shown in Figure 6.5.

A padded below knee cast incorporating the skeletal pin is sometimes used in conjunction with skeletal traction (Fig. 6.7). The mechanics of the traction are unchanged. The advantages of the cast are that the ankle is held in a good position while the calf is protected from compression between the edge of the sling and the skeletal pin. Movement of the pin is reduced to a minimum. This traction arrangement is also used in a fixed skeletal traction set-up (Charnley's traction unit) in the initial management of femoral shaft fractures.

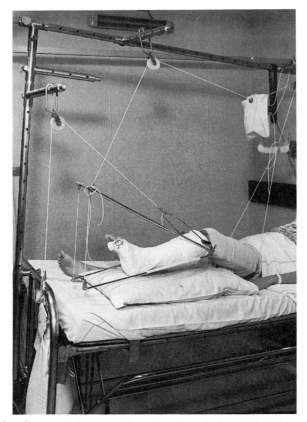

**Fig. 6.7** A below knee cast incorporating a traction pin inserted in the proximal tibia. Note that the suspension cords are not yet trimmed and taped so that final adjustment can be made to the suspension of the Thomas's splint.

### 2. Balanced skeletal traction in a Fisk splint

This splint allows active assisted flexion and extension of the hip and knee while traction is maintained. The Fisk splint consists of the upper part of a modified Thomas's splint attached to a knee flexion piece.

### 3. Balanced suspension in a Tulloch Brown splint

This splint is commonly used in adults to suspend the limb following pseudarthrosis surgery (Girdlestones operation), or following cap arthroplasty. The splint consists of a lightweight duralumin U-shaped loop with a pulley fixed to the distal end (Fig. 6.8). The side bars of the splint contain a series of holes to accommodate the ends of a skeletal pin at the appropriate level. The lower limb is cradled on supporting slings between the side bars of the splint.

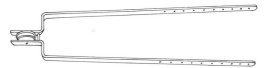

**Fig. 6.8** Tulloch Brown splint. Slings made of calico or flannel, or wide elastic tubular bandage can be placed on the sides of the loop to support the calf. The achilles tendon should be left free from pressure as shown in Figure 6.9.

The Tulloch Brown splint can be suspended using a single cord (Fig. 6.9) or by two separate cords and pulleys. The U-loop must lie evenly on either side of the leg. The sling under the calf must not compress the tissues between its edge and the skeletal pin. Check it regularly and loosen the sling if necessary. Countertraction is achieved by elevating the foot of the bed.

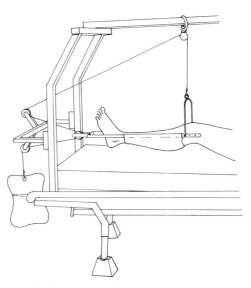

**Fig. 6.9** Balanced suspension in a Tulloch Brown splint. Careful observations are made to ensure that the tissues are not compressed between the upper edge of the sling supporting the leg and the rigid traction pin inserted in the proximal tibia.

### 4. Balanced vertical traction (90–90 traction)

This traction set-up (Fig. 6.10) is used in the management of femoral fractures in the subtrochanteric region which cannot be maintained in good alignment in a Thomas's splint. 90–90 traction allows good access to the posterior thigh if there is a wound to be managed, for example after a compound fracture. The hip and knee are flexed to 90°. The traction pull from the stirrup attached to the femoral or tibial

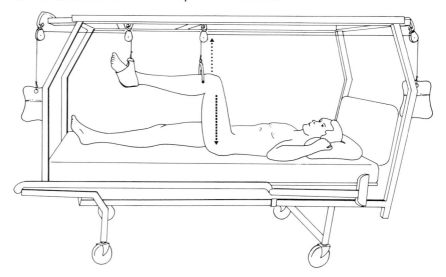

**Fig. 6.10** Balanced vertical traction (90–90 traction). The lower leg is suspended by means of a padded sling. This set up allows good access to the skin on the posterior thigh and calf. The heel should be inspected regularly for signs of pressure.

pin is vertical. Countertraction is provided by the weight of the patient's thigh. The lower leg can be supported by a:

a. sling
b. cast, incorporating a suspension hook
c. Tulloch Brown U-loop
d. skeletal pin in the lower tibia.

**Balanced traction in a Böhler-Braun frame.**

The thigh and lower leg are supported on slings between the side bars of the frame which rests on the bed. Pulleys are fixed to the Böhler-Braun frame to accommodate a traction cord from a distal femoral, proximal tibial, or a cancaneal pin. Countertraction is obtained by elevating the foot end of the bed. The leg rests on supporting slings which should be slack enough to avoid compressing the tissues of the calf. The patient's movements are more restricted by this type of suspension as the frame rests on the bed. However, the system is portable and, if necessary, the patient can be transported safely while in traction.

## COMPLICATIONS OF SKELETAL TRACTION

### 1. Infection

The insertion of a skeletal traction device inevitably results in some tissue reaction characterized by some serous drainage from the pin tract. The foreign body (pin or wire) remains in contact with the external environment and, therefore, there is a risk of contamination of the tissues adjacent to the pin or wire. This contamination usually remains inconsequential; however, certain factors will increase the chance of infection of the pin tract. These infections can lead to osteomyelitis, hence they must be avoided.

Redness and swelling around the pin site usually heralds the onset of infection. When a pin tract is infected, gentle percussion over the site of the bone through which the pin passes will be painful. The predisposing factors to pin site infection, apart from poor insertion technique, are:

(a) *Loosening of the pin or wire* which causes excessive movement between the pin and surrounding tissues. The pin or wire will need to be removed and an alternative site or mode of treatment instituted.

(b) *Tension of the skin and subcutaneous tissues* which can compromise the normal capillary blood flow leading to necrosis if unrelieved. Care must be taken to prevent compression of the tissues between the pin and the supporting slings of suspension apparatus. Obstruction of the drainage from the site will cause increased tension in the tissues and could lead to abscess formation. This can be avoided by cleaning the dried exudate away from the pin site and *gently* easing the tissue back from the pin if necessary.

Routine pin site management varies widely from hospital to hospital, and even within a ward according to physician preference. Whatever regime is followed, the technique should be aseptic and the incidence of pin tract infection closely monitored in each ward. If infections are occurring, the technique should be reviewed.

## 2. Overdistraction of the bone fragments

As a result of the heavy traction weights that can be used in skeletal traction, too much distraction can occur. Follow-up X-rays and limb length measurements are needed to check the position of the fracture as this complication can predispose to a delayed union or a non-union of the fracture.

## 3. Nerve damage

This can result from the use of heavy traction forces. Careful, regular assessment of nerve function (see Neurovascular Assessment, pp. 14–16) is mandatory and any deficit must be reported and acted upon at once.

## 4. Breaking of the pins or wire

Although unusual, this can occur particularly if the patient is very restless, for example following head injury, and heavy weights are used. In an instance such as this, the pin can be protected by incorporating it in a padded plaster cast as in Figure 6.7 (sometimes known as a Charnley traction unit).

REMOVAL OF SKELETAL TRACTION PINS

The type of pin used must be recorded in the patient's notes so that the correct technique is used to remove it. For example, a Steinmann's pin is simply pulled out, a Denham pin needs to be unscrewed until the threaded section is clear of the bone. Analgesia will need to be given with enough time allowed to elapse so that the patient gets the full benefit of it during removal of the Denham pin. The sharp end of the pin is thoroughly cleaned prior to removal. The pin is removed by gripping the blunt end with a chuck handle. Small depressed scars often remain at the pin hole sites. These scars are unsightly and unnecessary. They can be prevented by firmly pinching the pin tract at the time of removal of the pin. In this way the adhesion of the skin to the deeper tissues, due to fibrous tissue formation, is broken.

# Bibliography

**Brooker A F, Schmeisser G** 1980 Orthopedic traction manual. Williams and Wilkins, Baltimore

**Carini G K, Birmingham J** 1980 Traction made manageable: a self-learning module. McGraw-Hill, New York

**Farrell J** 1982 Illustrated guide to orthopedic nursing, 2nd edn. J B Lippincott, Philadelphia

**Hamilton Russell R** 1923–24 Fracture of the femur: a clinical study. British Journal of Surgery 11(43): 491–502

**Iverson L D, Clawson D K** 1982 Manual of acute orthopaedic therapeutics, 2nd edn. Little Brown and Company, Boston

Nursing Photobook™. Working with orthopedic patients. Nursing 84™. Pennsylvania's Springhouse Corporation

**Ogden J A** 1982 Skeletal injury in the child. Lea & Febiger, Philadelphia

**Powell M** 1986 Orthopaedic nursing and rehabilitation, 9th edn. Churchill Livingstone, Edinburgh

**Stewart J D M, Hallett J P** 1983 Traction and orthopaedic appliances, 2nd edn. Churchill Livingstone, Edinburgh

# Index